Marriage in
MODERN
Life

Dr. Anne Brennan Malec

Marriage in
MODERN
Life

WHY IT WORKS, WHEN IT WORKS

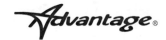

Published by Advantage, Charleston, South Carolina.
Member of Advantage Media Group.

ADVANTAGE is a registered trademark and the Advantage colophon is a trademark of Advantage Media Group, Inc.

Printed in the United States of America.

ISBN: 978-1-59932-528-6
LCCN: 2015939643

Book design by Megan Elger.

This publication is designed to provide accurate and authoritative information in regard to the subject matter covered. It is sold with the understanding that the publisher is not engaged in rendering legal, accounting, or other professional services. If legal advice or other expert assistance is required, the services of a competent professional person should be sought.

Advantage Media Group is proud to be a part of the Tree Neutral® program. Tree Neutral offsets the number of trees consumed in the production and printing of this book by taking proactive steps such as planting trees in direct proportion to the number of trees used to print books. To learn more about Tree Neutral, please visit www.treeneutral.com. To learn more about Advantage's commitment to being a responsible steward of the environment, please visit www.advantagefamily.com/green

Advantage Media Group is a publisher of business, self-improvement, and professional development books and online learning. We help entrepreneurs, business leaders, and professionals share their Stories, Passion, and Knowledge to help others Learn & Grow. Do you have a manuscript or book idea that you would like us to consider for publishing? Please visit advantagefamily.com or call 1.866.775.1696.

Few of us travel our road alone—and how much better that way. My sincere thanks to the following:

My teachers, Symmetry Counseling colleagues, siblings, friends, and—most especially—my clients, all of whom played a pivotal role in my personal and professional journey;

My colleague, Meghan Emerson, who joined me in the 18th mile of this marathon and ran with me to the finish line, providing critical insight and support;

The Malecs, who graciously welcomed me in 1995 as a family member, utterly enriching and broadening my life, providing love, humor, and the highs and lows experienced by every modern family;

My late father, Daniel Brennan, who passed along humor, candor, and a solid work ethic. My mother, Theresa Brennan, who continues to inspire me through love, faith, and smiling resilience; and

My husband, John, to whom I am so grateful for traveling with me not only on this journey of authorship but every other path we walk. He provided encouragement, support, keen editorial skill, and steadfast love. Always, for John.

TABLE OF CONTENTS

INTRODUCTION

As a clinical psychologist and a licensed marriage and family therapist, I founded Symmetry Counseling to assist couples and individuals struggling with life's pressures. Since 2011, the practice has grown from five therapists to thirty. Across the practice, our therapists lead thousands of sessions per year, and we see many unhappy people living in relationships that are not working.

A big factor in much of this unhappiness is that most of us were never prepared to succeed in our relationships. Unless you are in my field, your school curriculum touched only briefly on the topic or skipped it altogether. Further, key skills such as how to communicate, how to maintain a long-term relationship, and how to be a good partner are the focus of neither our upbringing nor our culture.

Consider the emphasis placed on the process of getting engaged and married versus how to successfully spend a lifetime together. Or consider the time and money spent on planning and having a wedding versus the perfunctory or nonexistent time spent in premarital counseling. This shows our priorities as a society. Many if not most couples enter into marriage with unrealistic expectations for what it will require from each partner to create a successful relationship. Many have the notion that when both parties say "I do," the hard part is over—that love is unconditional.

What you know about relationships you probably learned from your parents, extended family, friends, and your own trial and error. The most significant influence was probably your parents. Regardless of how well-meaning and loving your parents are, they probably learned the same way. They may not be able to pass on the skills you need today, or they may have actually passed along traits that are unhelpful. Friends are also well-intentioned. But those in happy relationships may talk little about "why." And from those whose relationships fail, you typically just hear how it was "all the other person's fault." Consequently, many people make the very significant commitment to a marriage or long-term relationship without any useful idea of what to expect—from themselves or their mates. All of us are constantly learning how to make our relationships work.

I was in the same boat. In my personal relationships, I made mistakes along the way. My parents' traditional marriage, with a strong patriarchal hand, was not a very useful model for helping me to succeed in a modern, 21st century marriage. Nor did it teach me how to be a stepmother to my husband's children.

When I married my husband nearly 16 years ago, I did not know what it would take to have a happy marriage. I was working in business and had not given much thought to how this new relationship and stepchildren were all going to work. What I knew about relationships, I had picked up from my parents and a religion class in college. I knew I loved my husband a lot and hoped life with him would be fun, interesting, and adventurous. Having earned an undergraduate degree in accounting, I knew a lot about business, but I had no formal education in how relation-ships work. While earning a master's degree in liberal studies from DePaul University, I enrolled in a class titled Resolving Conflicts in Organizations. It was in this class that I discovered my interest in the hows and whys of successful relationships. I continued my education by earning a graduate degree in marriage and family therapy from the Family Institute at Northwestern University. I later added a doctorate in clinical psychology from the Chicago School of Professional Psychology. But my most useful learning about relationships comes from observing and working with my clients, who daily share their stories and struggles with me.

In addition to a lack of training, I routinely note that people come to relationships with differing notions of "the rules." One of the assumed rules is that love is unconditional. Looking at the divorce rate, however, empirically love is one of the most conditional human activities. If unconditional to you means, "I will love you no matter what you do or how you treat me," your view is unrealistic. While we all have a good idea of the conditions under which we are willing to stay married, we give much less thought to the conditions under which our partner is willing to stay married to us.

The cultural belief that love is unconditional fosters the belief that marriage takes care of itself. In turn, this belief implies that succeeding in marriage or other long-term relationships does not take daily effort. The reality is that keeping a relationship alive and healthy requires a lot of "doing."

Married partners may not know how to fix their relationship, but we all know when things are heading in the wrong direction. The *most* common question I hear from couples that are trying to make it work is "How can we fix this?" If that is your purpose in reading this book, I am happy to offer you real hope. It is not magic. A successful relationship is built with dedication and effort and by fairly applying straightforward principles.

As a therapist, I have run into the same patterns couple after couple, year after year, and general principles and rules have evolved. I wrote this book to offer practical and actionable tools to help when problems arise. These tools have proven to help clients who are struggling with the pressures and expectations of modern marriage—pressures that only increase with the addition of a child or two. I am hopeful that these tools help you avoid emotional and physical disconnection caused by: poor communication; unmet and unreasonable expectations; and feeling unheard, neglected, and resentful. If you are already in conflict, it is my hope that these suggestions help you regain a balanced relationship.

To be useful, such tools need to be simple, straightforward, and, most importantly, fair. Perceived fairness is a vital component of a successful relationship. If one partner constantly feels overburdened, it can lead to relational burnout. If one partner is always stuck doing the heavy lifting, eventually it will lead to resentment and emotional disconnection. That is why this book is for both of you. Read it, discuss the suggestions, and apply them to your life together. Applying these principles will assist with maintaining a mutually beneficial relationship that becomes more binding than the "I do" you so hopefully declared early on.

CHAPTER ONE:

Marriage in Modern Life

Being part of a successful and loving relationship is one of the most rewarding aspects of life. If you asked random people what they most hoped to have in life, no doubt a joyful marriage would be among the top answers. If people crave a happy relationship, why do so many struggle and fail to maintain the relationship for a lifetime? Because it is not easy. Then again, few rewarding things in life are easy. During the early days and months of a relationship, known as the infatuation stage, partners can be under the false impression that a relationship will always be so effortless. But when infatuation inevitably diminishes and real life intrudes, your partner must remain a priority, or you will eventually run into trouble.

Your marriage is not guaranteed to work just because you had the right flowers and pretty bridesmaid dresses at your wedding. Your marriage does not fail because it rained on your wedding day, because the caterer overcooked the filet or because Uncle Al gave a hopelessly confused and inappropriate toast. Instead, most relationships succeed or fail based on joint commitment and the partners' relationship skills.

For many of us, relationship skills do not come naturally, and our relationship instincts are unrefined. Most partners use two learning strategies: (1) watching their parents and (2) trial and error.

One must be careful about applying too much truth to any one role model or relationship experience. Having parents, siblings, or friends whose relationship dissolved does not mean that your relationship is doomed to fail. The good news here is that being successful in your relationships does not require magic. Much of making a relationship work is a conscious choice—you and your partner control your destiny.

Relationships do not thrive because of luck or some secret formula but because the partners take actions that make their relationship a priority. The behaviors, skills, and attitudes you need can be learned. Do not think of it as work but as a necessary nurturing of your most valuable asset. You *can* develop the skills to succeed and thrive in your marriage, and it is never too late to learn. If you read this book and incorporate these suggestions in your marriage, you will be on a path to a healthier, more connected, and more rewarding relationship.

A CALL TO ACTION

Data collected from 2006 to 2010 indicate the failure rate of first-time marriages as follows: 20 percent fail within the first 5 years, 32 percent fail within the first 10 years, 40 percent fail within the first 15 years, and 48 percent fail within the first 20 years.[1] Divorced couples report the following reasons for the failure of their marriages: unmet emotional needs, lifestyle differences, boredom with the marriage, feeling demeaned within the relationship,[2] infidelity, incompatibility, drinking, drug use, poor communication skills, dissatisfaction with handling of joint financial issues, high levels of conflict, and young age at time of marriage.[3]

This data is consistent with what I have seen in my professional experience. Couples report experiencing ineffective and damaging communication patterns, more negative than positive interactions, and poor problem-solving skills. Partners also speak of unreasonable expectations, poor communication around finances, and a lack of prioritization of one's partner and the relationship. All of this creates disappointment or dissatisfaction that fosters resentment. Poor relationship habits lead to steady and persistent disconnection.

Many poor relationship habits stem from the false belief that marriage should not require work. The reasons for marrying in previous centuries arose from pragmatic needs: financial support, societal pressure, social standing, religion, procreation, or the merging of family interests. But today, marriage is romanticized as a choice made solely out of love. Our culture perpetuates the fantasy of the *happily-ever-after marriage*, where newlyweds ride off into the sunset and go on to achieve their house with a white picket fence and 2.5 kids. It may seem unromantic to view love as a thing that can slip through the grasp of partners who do not actively nurture each other and the relationship, but fantasy is not reality. Marriage is not an automatic happily-ever-after but a journey toward fulfillment that requires active participation by both parties.

A relationship, like everything we value, is not self-sustaining. It requires frequent attention and effort. An intimate relationship is a living, breathing organism that requires nurturing, feeding, and care. Why do people lose sight of this? Because human beings have the tendency to get used to all that is good in their lives; that is, we habituate. The people with whom we were at one time completely smitten begin to lose a bit of their sheen when we spend all of our time with them. Without the spark of new love, a relationship becomes one of the competing demands in your life. All of us are guilty of this natural phenomenon, and we are all responsible for increasing our awareness and keeping our relationships interesting.

When first dating my husband, I recall telling my sister that I could not imagine a time when I would no longer have lunch with him every day, but fast-forward 20 years, I realized one day while driving home from the office that I had not communicated with him since 7:30 that morning. Over time, we become susceptible to taking our partners for granted; we cease to treat them as we did when we first met and began to spend time together. They become very familiar. Familiarity brings us comfort and a sense of safety, but it also drains novelty, which relationships need.

Society's obsession with technology, such as computers, video games, and smartphones, is a modern symptom of the human desire for novelty and distraction. Technology competes with and often wins our attention away from our partners and family. Head to a restaurant or movie theater, and I guarantee you will find a couple where one or both partners peruse their phones instead of directly interacting with one another. We are all susceptible to the distractions available through technology because it provides sufficient stimulation with little effort on our part. Sometimes we are distracted by world events that deserve our attention, but more often our relationships simply do not measure up to the diversion acquired through technology. In long-term relationships, many partners gradually become unwilling to expend the extra effort it takes to create novelty with their spouses. However, this was not always the case in most relationships. Partners can usually think back to a time near the beginning of a relationship when their new love interest was the sole distraction and fulfilled all needs for diversion and novelty.

If you are reading this book, you have probably felt the completely delightful experience of falling in love. Our bodies and brains overwhelm us, intoxicating us with hormones and neurotransmitters that mimic an addiction to our partners. The infatuation stage is the period where people are likely to talk about their "soul mates" and view the relationship as infallible. Inevitably, that head-over-heels, obsessive kind of love lessens over time. In the best relationships, infatuation matures to a much deeper attachment. In a very real sense, it becomes true love. You might not have butterflies anymore, but you have consistency, reliability, and trust—a close friendship based on shared feelings and experiences. You know without conscious thought that this person has your best interests in mind, just as you have theirs. Even though your body chemistry is no longer hyper-focused on your beloved, your relationship still requires the level of nurturing and personal attention you gave so easily in the early phases. In fact, when a deeper connection develops, that is your call to action to maintain those physical and emotional intimacies that help your relationship thrive.

The modern marriage has the complicating challenge of managing the human tendency to habituate with our desire for relationship security, novelty, and excitement. A tall order, indeed. We become attracted to our partners and establish a monogamous relationship, but then we get used to them and take them for granted. We do not see them through fresh eyes and gradually lessen the effort we put forth to make our partners feel special. But your partner liked feeling they were the center of your universe and will not like feeling that they have fallen off the pedestal.

It feels great to feel special, right? And it hurts to feel less than special. Your mate felt special because you made him or her feel that way. When you stop, your partner will notice. You need to continue purposefully to care and to nurture each other.

Consistent friendship, steadfast support, and mutual trust may not sound rip-your-clothes-off exciting, but it is worth prioritizing and cherishing. When something good happens, you want someone you can call and know that he or she will be happy for you. You want a partner to have your back when you take a calculated business risk. You want him or her to pick you up when you feel sad. You want a partner to encourage you when you have self-doubt. You want a partner to love you, even if you fail or show some of your bad qualities (and we all have them). You want loyalty and respect, which is what you hear again and again from people who have been married a long time: "We're friends. We look after each other. We care about each other. We can tell when the other one is feeling down." The greater focus you put toward creating a solid marital bond built from mutual support and respect, healthy and frequent communication, and steady and frequent expressions of affection, the stronger foundation you have to handle life's ups and downs, including the transition to parenthood.

Children are a common excuse used by unhappy couples as to why there is not enough time or energy to devote to the relationship. The marital happiness curve theory postulates a U-shaped curve of marital satisfaction that starts high at the honeymoon period, drops abruptly with the birth of children, and then climbs after all children have left the nest. This well-researched pattern reveals that children take a significant toll on marital happiness.[4] As any parent knows, children bring another conflicting set of needs into play. It is understandable how and why many couples place their marriages on the back burner to attend to the needs of their children. However, this cannot be your long-term strategy, as you may eventually find your marriage in tatters. I know of no marriage that can survive with an excessive backlog of deferred marital maintenance.

Often couples I see tell me, "I thought that once the kids grow up, we would reconnect." Perhaps, but it is risky to rely solely on this expectation. Modern society pressures partners to give themselves to their children ahead of all other relationships and priorities. When you are focusing all of your efforts, attention, love, and affection on your children, the parents' relationship can wither and die. Feeling busy, tired, and guilty for not spending more time with your kids is the norm for many couples. However, try not to lose sight of the fact that in addition to you and your partner, your children are also the beneficiaries of a loving and nurtured marriage. Remember that you are teaching them how to have a good marriage.

Our culture venerates families but may not paint an accurate picture of the realities of married life with children. If you allow your marriage to become less important than your children, years later, when the kids have launched, you may not *know* each other anymore. This potential reality reminds me of a scene from the movie *About Schmidt.* Jack Nicholson, playing a longtime married man nearing retirement and reflecting on his life, looks at his wife and thinks, "Who is this old woman who lives in my house?"[5] So funny yet so accurate. There is so much professional, personal, and emotional growth that goes on individually over the decades of parenting that spouses can almost become strangers who are just coparenting. Such a relational dynamic is susceptible to unhappiness, resentment, emotional and physical disconnection, and infidelity.

While time together yields shared experiences, memories, and closeness, it takes more to sustain a satisfying relationship. It is also important to keep yourself interesting and attractive to your mate. After the infatuation period wears off, every relationship is at risk of becoming susceptible to a "sameness" of being with one person day in and day out. The "sameness" can lead to increasing boredom with you, your partner, and the relationship. Keep it fresh and be both interesting to yourself and to your partner. Marriage is not just a ceremony or event; it is a long-term commitment that needs your attention and investment, just like your car requires gas. Do not expect your relationship to run indefinitely on fumes. As Clint Black sings, "Love isn't something that we find, it's something that we do."[6]

It is not uncommon for both men and women to feel dissatisfaction due to a decline in positive behaviors after marriage. Partners often reduce the frequency or altogether stop doing the things that caused the other to fall in love with them. Knowledge is power: it does not have to be this way if you do not want it to be.

Marriage is a long-term investment. It is an asset—perhaps your most important asset—that you want to protect, grow, and develop. Your relationship requires frequent deposits; without those deposits, your relationship will atrophy. Answer the call to action, and begin fortifying and enhancing your modern marriage.

═══ POINTS TO REMEMBER ═══

- Make your partner and your relationship a priority.

- Making your marriage work is a choice, and it requires *work*.

- Make the effort to learn the skills that support a successful marriage.

- Keep yourself, and therefore your relationship, fresh and interesting.

- Show daily affection in the form of hugs and kisses.

- Express daily gratitude for your spouse—thank them for something they did.

- Compliment your spouse.

- Give your partner some of your undivided, screen-free attention every day.

For more helpful resources, go to:
www.DrAnneMalec.com

CHAPTER TWO:

Communication
Is the Oxygen

A lot of things about marriage and relationships have changed since our parents' day, beginning with communication. Most of us learned about marriage and how it worked (or did not work) from watching our parents. My mother's work was largely done in the home, raising a large brood of children and spearheading community volunteer programs. My father was the breadwinner and got the final vote on most of the big family decisions.

My parents' traditional relationship style was more the rule than the exception for that generation. This traditional relationship model is very clear about who is responsible for each task required to keep a family functioning. My parents rarely asked questions about or discussed whose role it was to get up during the night for a crying baby, cook dinner, do the laundry, or make the major financial decisions for the family. I surmise that frequent communication about these types of family issues was not required because the roles were firmly established, and it went without saying how responsibilities were shared. However, fewer modern relationships embrace that traditional model, with more couples striving to achieve an equal partnership.

Many of us did not see our parents communicate about the issues that need discussing in a modern relationship, so new and more equitable ways of engaging and interacting with our partners may not come naturally. The good news is that it is never too late to create a relational style that meets the needs of the 21st century family—a style that is mutually beneficial and emotionally rewarding and in which responsibility, accountability, and decision-making are shared.

Communication in a relationship works like oxygen, sustaining life. Couples never come into my office and say, "We are talking way too much." It is always, "We have a problem with communication." I rarely take that to mean the partners are not talking, and I understand the subtext signifies that they are not *successfully* communicating. It may mean that one or both partners backs away from communication or limits their conversation to the unimportant things. Perhaps past conversations between the two became heated and escalated to the point that someone got angry or shut down. For many of us, our natural instinct is to avoid situations that feel complicated and confrontational. But keeping and maintaining a successful marriage depends on learning how to fight the "avoidance" instinct effectively and discussing difficult issues.

The only way to keep the lines of communication open is to make the talking space emotionally safe. Both partners in the relationship need to know that their concerns, feelings, anxieties, complaints, plans, and dreams will be heard respectfully. Being married for 16 years, I know this is easier said than done. It is not easy to listen to your partner when you are completely opposed to or misunderstand his or her perspective. It is not easy, but communication works best if you come to the discussion table with an open, patient, and tolerant mind. If emotional safety is lacking and if partners do not feel as though they can be honest and emotionally vulnerable, yet nonetheless heard—then they will likely back away from the interaction, physically or emotionally. To be able to share openly with a partner, one must know he or she will not be yelled at, belittled, dismissed, invalidated, rejected, or ignored.

Couples who fall into bad relationship habits that cut off communication comprise a significant portion of my practice. Typically, one spouse brings up a sensitive topic or maybe even a seemingly ordinary one, like getting help with the kids while he or she cooks dinner. The responding spouse may react poorly or not at all to the request, which then causes the initiating spouse to feel dismissed, frustrated, and resentful. Often the initiating spouse then shuts down and stops trying to communicate because doing so seems to have made things worse.

If you avoid difficult conversations and conflict because you fear that it will turn ugly, you need to get help with that issue unless you have a partner who is also conflict-avoidant. Two conflict-avoidant people can successfully navigate a relationship only if you both are truly willing to let things roll off your back and not secretly build resentment. But even then, it would benefit your relationship if you worked on building your conversational muscles. It never hurts to become a better communicator.

If you have chosen a partner who is not conflict-avoidant, who values communicating about small and large issues, and you are conflict avoidant, you potentially have trouble. Even if you are successful at avoiding verbal communication, you still communicate behaviorally. In my field we call this being passive-aggressive; that is, acting out your feelings instead of talking about them. As a relationship strategy, passive-aggression ranks near the bottom because of the mixed messages it sends. You say one thing but do another, or worse, you say nothing but roll your eyes or sigh dramatically. This interaction style communicates judgment and contempt, which is disrespectful and hurtful to your partner. It also dramatically lessens the likelihood that you will feel heard or understood by your partner.

When we act passive-aggressively, we usually do so because discussing our thoughts, feelings, and opinions with our partner makes us uncomfortable or seems too risky. I see it all the time in my practice: a partner agrees to do something when he or she has no intention of doing it, just so the spouse will stop nagging about it. For example, a partner conveniently "forgets" about a social commitment because he does not want to go but found it difficult to tell his wife how he felt. Another example: a partner who is afraid of telling her spouse that she finds him controlling acts out her feelings by arriving home three hours later than she had agreed to and blaming her phone's battery for not being able to call him. Passive-aggressive habits create distance between partners and may lead to resentment, emotional and physical disconnection, and marital distress.

Another common unhealthy communication dynamic is the partner who chooses not to communicate needs or desires verbally because he or she expects the other partner just to *know*. This person may believe, "If my partner loves me, he or she will know what I need or want." Expecting your partner to know intuitively what you want without saying it sets your partner up to fail. None of us are mind readers. Test yourself: look at your spouse right now and determine what he or she is thinking, feeling, or needing. How did you do? Probably not well. It is far more effective—and you stand the best chance of getting your needs met—if you learn to share your thoughts directly with your partner.

Be especially alert to the relationship danger in wanting your partner to know what you want or need when you do not even know it yourself. It is a very childish relationship game: guess what I need or want, and I will tell you if it feels right. By playing this game, you risk setting yourself up to be disappointed and blaming your partner for failing at a game he or she could not possibly win.

How do we structure our relationship in a way that makes communicating information, opinions, feelings, concerns, and disappointments more likely to head off problems instead of cause them? I encourage my clients to have at least a 20-minute daily check-in and also to have a weekly meeting with a specific agenda. Every couple needs this daily screen-free time to catch up on the events of the day and talk about what is coming up the following day (this can make for smoother mornings in getting yourselves and the kids out of the house).

It is paramount that daily check-ins and weekly meetings remain free of technological distraction. The invasion of technology into modern life, which has brought with it tremendous benefits and ease of communication, has also negatively affected our intimate relationships. Researchers found "the mere presence of mobile phones inhibited the development of interpersonal closeness and trust and reduced the extent to which individuals felt empathy and understanding from their partners... These effects are most pronounced if individuals were discussing a personally meaningful topic."[7] Additionally, in a 2014 survey, 70 percent of women reported that "technoference"[8] was interfering in their romantic relationships. Technoference is defined as daily "intrusions or interruptions in couple interactions or time spent together…due to technology." Those reporting technoference also reported more conflict over technology use, lower relationship satisfaction, more depressive symptoms, and lower life satisfaction. While these findings are impressive, more astounding (evoking quite an image) is the report that 10 percent of cell phone users admit to using their phones during sex.[9] This data suggests that couples today need firm boundaries and rules about the use of technology so it does not interfere with their relationship. In my practice, couples commonly resist the idea of leaving their cell phones out of reach when at home. However, doing so is a simple way of telling your partner that you are present and available for interactions. (Clients will often apologize to me for any phone activity during a session; I wonder if they also apologize to their partners for the same inattentiveness.)

Many partners report that after the kids are in bed, they are both so drained from the day that they go to their separate corners and do their own thing. This "own thing" can be watching TV, playing video games, reading, or surfing the Internet, to name a few. I know that you are tired, but sitting and talking to your partner about your day should be restorative, not exhausting. Some days you may do more listening then talking, but such time is critical to a couple's long-term connection.

As mentioned previously, another way to stay connected and keep lines of communication healthy and functioning is by scheduling weekly check-in meetings with your spouse to discuss bigger picture items that you may not have time to thoughtfully discuss on a daily basis. Such issues might include financial or work goals, parenting concerns, concerns about household division of labor, or issues that are troubling you. Some couples may do better with an agenda communicated beforehand. Many couples do fine with a spoken agenda, but more conflict-ridden couples may require a written agenda to keep them focused and the conversation running smoothly. If one partner is unwilling to discuss an agenda item at the proposed time, he or she needs to propose an alternate time and stick to it so as to respect the other partner's needs. Partners can become frustrated when a discussion gets delayed, so do youself and your partner a favor by meeting your self-imposed deadline. This will build trust and limit resentment.

How formal should the agenda and discussion be? It depends on the couple. Couples needing more structure might consider using a clock to ensure there is equal talking time. Partners can usc an object like a spoon or book that is passed back and forth to indicate who is the speaker to keep themselves centered and reduce the likelihood of either partner becoming overheated. The purpose of the meeting is to focus on the issues at hand but not revisit past arguments or disappointments. If you find yourself becoming angry at your partner or either of you going on tangents unrelated to present circumstances, it is wise to provide more structure to the meetings that limit such tendencies. If you are having trouble agreeing on how to discipline or talk to your children or what parenting rules to apply—that is what the agenda topic should be. It should not be allowed to morph into "Well, you're spending too much money" or "Your whole family is like this."

The beauty about having weekly meetings is that each partner knows that no matter how busy you both are, you have this time scheduled to address concerns or frustrations. It does not have to be a sit-down meeting at the dining table, either. Maybe it is when you walk the dog or go out for dinner; maybe it is in the morning sharing coffee before the kids get up or when you meet for lunch. Just set a mutually agreed upon time when you can get together and talk. It is important that you make it a priority—something that you both consciously schedule—rather than waiting for it to occur on its own. If it is not scheduled, it probably will not happen.

WE NEED TO TALK: What do you discuss at your weekly check-in meetings? Typical topics might include: the upcoming week's schedule; the needs and schedules of the children; who is in charge of planning date night for the week; perceived fairness of the household division of labor; upcoming travel or social plans; agreeing on family or individual expenses; issues that need problem-solving or brainstorming; and either party's current worries, concerns, or stresses.

Think of this scheduled time as relationship muscle building. It serves as a means of prioritizing the couple, and every relationship needs to feel valued. I cannot overstate the importance of relationship self-care. Find what works best in terms of where and when, but whatever that best time and place is, be sure it is on both of your calendars. It is also important that you put a time limit on the scheduled conversation, even setting a timer if necessary, and that each person has a specified portion of that time. In this way, you are setting the agenda, carving out a time slot, and reassuring your partner that no, this conversation will not go on all night and stray into every possible area (you can always add time later if issues remain unresolved). If you set a timer for 20 or 30 minutes, you might not get very far in the conversation, but it builds skill and discipline, as well as respect. Knowing that each partner will have the floor at some point keeps you from feeling like you need to lob comments at the other quickly before one of you storms out of the room. A scheduled, shared, regular communication session can go a long way toward being successful in communicating about difficult things. Other ground rules: using a respectful tone of voice and no yelling, sarcasm, or dismissiveness.

As important as verbal communication is, sometimes partners do not want to talk immediately about things as they occur. Some people prefer to sort things out mentally before discussing an issue. I have found this to be especially true for many men. If you sense that your husband is struggling with something, and you ask him about it, let it be okay if he does not want to get into it with you in the moment. Men do not always benefit from airing their troubles like women do. That is okay; there is nothing wrong with it—it is just a different way of processing. Providing temporary space is not meant to excuse men from discussing a topic indefinitely. Communicate with your partner about how much time you need on your own before discussing it together, and agree on a time that is comfortable for both of you. For the female partner, find a way to express your interest in discussing a topic while still allowing your spouse the flexibility he needs to feel ready. One suggestion: invite your partner by saying, "It is important to me that we find the time to discuss X. Please let me know if today or tomorrow evening works better for you. If neither of those times are good for you, please suggest a couple others."

Particularly when beginning a discussion, it is very important to introduce a topic or invite your spouse to a discussion in a manner that is welcoming and unthreatening. If there are difficult or sensitive feelings that you need to communicate, say something like, "Here's how I felt in this situation. It would feel better to me if it were handled differently in the future." Then suggest how you would prefer it be handled, making sure to suggest differences for yourself in addition to what your partner should do differently.

The subtext here is: I feel this way, and I want to feel better, so can changes be made so I can feel better? Keep the focus on coming up with ideas to solve the problem. And remember, just because one of you feels a certain way about something does not mean that your partner caused that feeling. All kinds of things happen in life without it being the specific fault of anyone. Avoid sweeping generalizations, such as:

- "You never see my side."
- "You always just dismiss me."
- "You always pick your family over me."
- "You never listen to me."

Even if some part of you feels that is the case, generalizations that include "always" and "never" are (almost) never true. Statements like these make the other person defensive and angry, and your partner may feel driven to point out any and every exception to your statement rather than listening to and addressing your feelings. Avoid insulting terms, name calling, or swearing. It is not necessary, it will not get your point across, and it will only anger the other.

The more accurately you state your concerns or complaints, the more effective you will be in making yourself heard. Never threaten divorce in the midst of a fight; avoid statements such as "I am done with this" or "I am done with you." It is scary and threatening and can lead to unintended consequences. You are allowed to feel strongly about an issue, but communicating in a calm, straightforward manner that acknowledges the likelihood that your partner feels differently gives you the best chance of having your needs addressed.

Although it can be easy to veer off topic, it is important to stick to the agenda. If you feel as though your partner said something that is unfair, out of context, or spiteful, try to let it pass and bring the discussion back on topic. In every marriage, there are going to be issues that require bringing all your maturity, patience, and caring to the situation at hand. A lot can go wrong when you talk about the tough stuff—but much more can go wrong if you avoid it.

Once the discussion starts, if one or both of you feel as though you are getting worked up, call a halt to the conversation. You know when you start to lose your cool: your breathing changes, your heart beats a little faster, your face gets hot, and your brain becomes flooded with thoughts and feelings. You stop listening because you cannot wait for the other person to stop talking so you can make your point. Once someone has started to get over-heated or angry, the conversation has gone off the rails. Nothing good comes from continuing then and there. Anger can feel good to the brain. It is an adrenaline rush and often feels empowering. Watch out for this. When you notice anger building, say something like, "Okay, this isn't going very well, and I'm starting to lose it, so let's try it again tomorrow. Same time, same place." The essential piece is to reschedule it right then and not let it slide. For the non-angry partner, it can feel very frustrating when the discussion gets halted. However, view your partner asking for the time as an attempt to protect the relationship (and you) from his or her anger getting out of control.

If you find that this often happens, that one or both of you gets overheated when you are trying to hash out a problem, you might consider trying the speaker/listener technique. Implementing this approach helps to slow things down and reduces the likelihood of reactionary comments. The guidelines are as follows: Each member of the couple takes turns speaking and listening in the meeting. The partner with an issue begins as the speaker, expressing his or her feelings in two to three sentences. The listener paraphrases the speaker's message and is only allowed to ask questions for clarification. The speaker does not turn over his or her role as speaker until the listener conveys a thorough understanding of what the speaker is trying to say. Once the speaker feels heard, he or she becomes the listener, and the former listener now has an opportunity to respond to the original speaker's comments. The discussion continues in this manner until both partners reach a solution. Partners must agree not to speak over each other. If one partner gets upset and feels a need to call a halt to the meeting, he or she does so for an agreed upon period.

For example, a wife might say "I get very angry when you say you're going to get home from work by 6:30. I plan the evening and get dinner ready, and then you text me at 6:45 saying, 'Something came up, I'm not going to be home until 8:00.' That is very upsetting to me." In his role as the listener, the husband will restate what his wife said: "What you are saying is, you get upset when I've promised to be home at a particular time, and you have planned accordingly, then I call to say I will be late." Ideally, the husband does not become defensive or start explaining, rationalizing, or attacking his wife's feelings. When the wife feels that the husband interpreted her correctly, they switch roles. As the speaker, the husband might respond, "I am sorry I have not been reliable in the past and miscommunicated when I would be home. That is disrespectful of you. Maybe in the future I can communicate earlier if I find that I am going to be home later than expected because a meeting is running long." The focus shifts from "you did something wrong" to "how should we develop a system that works better for both of us in this particular situation?" I realize that the speaker/listener technique can feel corny or somewhat awkward to people, but it is very effective in slowing down the conversation and allowing each partner to feel heard. It may not be a long-term solution, but it is a beneficial temporary exercise that allows both partners the opportunity to develop healthier communication skills.

Again, the goal is to *slowwwww it down*. The piece where you let your partner know you have heard and understood what is being said is an important aspect of healthy communication that often goes missing in everyday conversation. If you are truly listening to your partner, it naturally slows down the interaction. When truly listening to another, we are focused only on what he or she is saying rather than on what to say in response.

Slowing things down lessens the risk of escalation, which reduces the chance of getting conversationally derailed. Continuing a derailed argument will not allow you to reach the outcome you were hoping for unless your goal was for both of you to become mad and hurt.

There are times when you may feel so overwhelmed that you need to physically leave the room in order to marshal your feelings and not lose your cool. It is okay to take a time-out, but do not just get up and walk out without saying anything. Speak as calmly as you can, and say something along the lines of, "Listen, I'm getting flooded, and I don't want to say something stupid that I'm going to regret tomorrow. So I'm going to stop this now because I'm getting angry, and I'm not feeling heard." Avoid using provocative language in your request, like "You are not listening to me" or "You are a jerk." Take ownership of your need to pause the conversation, and remain respectful of your partner.

The reason to take a time-out is because the body's physiological response to getting agitated, angry, and flooded can cause the thinking part of the brain to go offline. Respect that the body has gotten worked up and that it needs time to settle down. Some people find taking a 30-minute walk helps them get back in control of their emotions. Others can feel better after a good night's sleep or from time spent cleaning a room, meditating, reading, listening to music, working on a project, or exercising. If your partner needs space and wants to call a stop to your discussion, you need to grant that request. Make a rule ahead of time that limits time-outs to lasting no more than 24 hours. That gives the angry partner time to calm down and think clearly about what set him or her off. It also reassures the other partner that the discussion will still be had.

If your partner walks out of the room to seek personal space, do not chase after him or her. Leave your partner alone until he or she is feeling calmer. Pursuing an angry partner who needs distance will only serve to escalate further and derail your conversation. Give your partner time to cool down and wait until he or she is ready to talk. A note to the withdrawing partner: it is very important that you return to the discussion when you are feeling in better control of your thoughts and emotions. Otherwise, you run the risk of your partner feeling like he or she has to chase you when you seek distance. Time-outs are only effective when the partner needing space feels that he or she is free to take it and the other partner feels reassured that the conversation will eventually continue.

In addition to structuring your discussions to limit the likelihood of emotional escalation, it is important to beware of common unhealthy communication habits. Let me speak again on the problem of expecting our mates to know our wants and needs intuitively: "Why can't he see that the garbage needs to be taken out?" Or, "Why can't she see that I'm tired?" When you expect your partner to *know what to do or how you feel*, you expect your mate to see through your eyes—and your partner cannot because he or she is not you. When we were infants incapable of communicating with words, we relied on our caregivers to intuitively sense our needs. But at that point in life, our needs were simple and most often related to hunger, cleanliness, sleep, and security. As adults, our needs are far more complex; we require understanding, empathy, nurturing, affection, validation, emotional support, problem solving, advice, and so on. It is your responsibility to let your spouse know about your needs, because no one's spouse is a mind reader.

Other ineffective communication habits I commonly see in my practice include the tester and the silent treatment. The spouse who sets up "tests" to see how much his or her partner cares about him or her often carries buried insecurities. Tests may be about remembering something specific, like a birthday gift or a favorite meal. The testing spouse might secretly tally who says "I love you" first, how quickly his or her partner responds to a text message, or how long his or her partner goes without initiating sex or giving affection. Isn't it more effective to tell your partner how you are feeling and what you need? If you find that you are putting your partner through a "test," realize that you are trying to find ways that he or she is failing you. When we look for ways to be disappointed, we usually find them.

The silent treatment is also an ineffective way to send a message and is often a form of passive aggression. Perhaps you have experienced it yourself: You ask your partner what is bothering her, and she says, "nothing," but her body language and all the cabinet-slamming says something completely different. Maybe the angry spouse is uncomfortable with confrontation and wants his or her partner to guess at what is wrong, so chooses to act out feelings instead of verbalizing them. Whatever your reason for not talking about your upset feelings, if you want your partner to know what is bothering you, you need to share it and acknowledge the negative emotion within yourself. Playing a guessing game or sulking only serves to frustrate both of you and creates emotional distance. Take the chance to tell your partner how you feel about what he or she did. It helps if you can do so respectfully, remaining mindful of your tone of voice and taking ownership of your feelings ("*I* feel frustrated that you have not applied for a job yet" instead of "*You* are being lazy and need to get a job"). Communicating our likes, dislikes, needs, and desires is crucial in a marriage.

Healthy couple communication is not just about effectively expressing your needs but also about being an active listener and desiring to understand your partner's perspective. Try not to blame your partner when you act on assumptions rather than seeking to understand his or her point of view. An example of this occurred years ago before I became a therapist. It was my husband's, John's, birthday, and I wanted to make him a chocolate cake, which is my favorite dessert. I thought he would love it because, well, I love it. And so I made him the cake from scratch (even the frosting), seeking out a special recipe. When he came home from playing golf that afternoon, I made a big fuss over all I did on his behalf, how I made this cake just for him, and surely he was so grateful. To my confusion and disappointment, he said, "Well, all I wanted for my birthday was for you to come out and play golf with me." He did not want the chocolate cake; he wanted me to spend time with him on his birthday. I never asked him how he wanted to celebrate his day.

That example shows that what we think makes another happy is often based on what makes us happy. This assumption can be especially risky between partners because we quite often have different needs and wishes. I gave John what I would have wanted for myself instead of asking him what he wanted. Lesson learned. (For a quick way to assess how you and your partner best receive love, take the quiz at www.5lovelanguages.com.)[10]

If you do not listen well or make efforts to understand your partner's perspective, your partner will not feel safe expressing his or her needs. The components of respectful listening are:

- Being patient as your partner articulates his or her thoughts and feelings.

- Waiting until you know your partner has fully expressed him or herself before paraphrasing and sharing your response.

- Trying to put yourself in his or her shoes (I know this is tough, but it creates a more empathic experience).

- Maintaining solid eye contact.

- Not exhibiting any nonverbal signs of disagreement or frustration, such as eye rolls, checking the time, looking at your phone, deeply exhaling, head shaking, or inappropriate laughter.

Being a respectful listener also means being attentive to how you respond to your partner. When you respond, be mindful of:

- Keeping a moderate tone of voice.

- Not yelling.

- Not being accusatory or talking over your partner.

- Accepting your partner's feelings and not saying how you think he or she is wrong, stupid, misguided, nonsensical, irrational, or crazy.

Negative responses invalidate your partner's needs and feelings. Invalidation is dangerous because you are telling your partner that he or she is *wrong* to think or feel that way. It is hurtful and pro-foundly disrespectful because everyone's feelings are very real to them. You need to work hard at validating, even if you disagree. Realize that even though you may have a difference of opinion and perspective, it does not mean that your partner is *wrong*; it just means that your opinions and perspectives are *different*. Tell your partner that you are having a hard time understanding because you view the situation so differently. Own your feelings of frustration and avoid putting unnecessary blame on your partner's valid perspective.

Sharing a different opinion or perspective should not be perceived as a lack of love. Strong initial reactions by one or both of you may be a reaction to fear or anxiety, which can be lessened by increased conversation and understanding. Both of you have the responsibility to bring structure, listening skills, and emotional self-soothing to the discussion table. If you do not practice these skills, discussions lead to arguments, which lead to chronic escalation and unresolved issues and ultimately resentment or emotional shutdown.

And do not rush to give advice, particularly if you have not been asked for it. You may presume that when your spouse is pouring out his or her heart to you about a problem, he or she is looking to you to fix it—but that is not necessarily the case. If instead of just respectfully listening to your partner, you launch into, "Well, here's what I'd do," he or she may get irritated, because advice may not be what is needed in the moment. Offering advice without being asked for it can feel insensitive and invalidating. Sometimes listening means just listening and not solving. Each of you should get into the habit of telling your partner when you want him or her to listen or to help problem-solve, which is a simple but highly effective strategy for feeling heard and supported.

TOUGH STUFF: Some subjects are naturally more difficult for people to talk openly about. Here is a list—by no means exhaustive—of topics that might require extra sensitivity and care:

- Spending, saving, investing
- Levels of affection and sex
- Physical health of your partner
- Emotional health concerns like depression or anxiety
- In-law and stepchildren conflicts
- Childcare responsibilities
- Household division of labor
- Parenting styles

Effective listening also means allowing your partner to finish a thought, sentence, or paragraph. Talking over or interrupting the other is a common problem with couples. The disrespectful behavior may stem from a fear of being misunderstood, but this communication style can lead to a dysfunctional cycle where one partner gets frustrated and determines that it is not worth the effort. Has your partner ever turned to you with complete exasperation and said irritably, "Will you *please* let me finish?" You run the risk of shutting down open communication when you fail to give your partner the space to verbally communicate, by telling your partner how he or she feels or thinks, by cutting your partner off, or by telling your partner that he or she is wrong. There is little incentive to communicate if one feels that his or her partner does not want to listen. If you feel like you need more structure to keep the discussion focused and your conversation space effective, make it a habit to ask your partner if he or she is finished speaking or utilize the speaker/listener technique described previously.

Some things are easier to talk about or listen to than others, but no topic should be classified as off-limits simply because one of you wants it to be so. Avoidance or denial does not make a problem go away; it just keeps simmering in the background until it bubbles over and burns both of you. If a partner is uncomfortable with certain topics or resists open discussion of them, consider limiting the time spent on them, say 20 minutes, with follow-ups as needed. Some topics require short, scheduled conversations over days, months, or years. There are some topics about which you and your partner may never completely agree or see eye to eye. That is okay; this is normal for most couples. The important thing is to revisit these points of disagreement now and then to see if there has been a change in perspective. Many issues between couples are not of critical importance and do not need immediate resolution. For other points of difference, complete resolution may not be required at all. We are all individuals, and that is what the term means. Some long-term points of difference will flare up occasionally, but it does not mean that your relationship is fatally flawed. We often change our minds as we age; issues that had at one time been deal-breakers can become less important over time.

Individual life dreams are one of these things that can require discussions over many years. Just because you have a dream does not make it your partner's dream. Do not try to guilt, steamroll, or manipulate your way into getting your partner to buy into your dream, as it is a short-term solution to a longer-term problem and will create resentment. The partner with a life-changing dream must be able to hear that his or her partner probably has a different dream that is equally valid to his or her own. Bring your willingness to compromise: hardly any of us gets exactly what we want 100 percent of the time. Can you live with 75 percent? Is 50 percent okay?

If you want your partner to feel comfortable sharing his or her life dreams and goals with you (and it is important that he or she does so and feels emotionally safe in doing so), it is essential that you be willing to hear your partner fully. Create a safe conversational space and do not shoot down or poke holes in the ideas prematurely. Invite the partner with the life-changing dream to explain how he or she thinks it will work. If it concerns a change in where you will live, for instance, have your partner discuss how you will both earn a living. Can children and family visit easily, and can you work in a foreign country without a visa? Sometimes the dream is just that, a dream. In the light of day, it will be hard to achieve, but it is still okay to talk about it.

Every couple may have issues that the partners cannot resolve no matter how frequently they try to discuss them. At times like this I hope you will consider going to work with a marriage and family therapist (MFT). MFTs are trained to assist couples struggling with the more complex issues of marriage, like communication styles, money, sexual/intimacy differences, children, in-laws, household division of labor, trust, and substance and behavioral addictions. A third party can bring a fresh perspective that cannot always be achieved by the couple.

You never want to reach the point where either one of you feels as though "We don't talk about it well, so we're not going to talk about it at all." If this is how you feel, then you need to see a therapist. A skilled clinician can help you have that discussion and teach you some of the skills that I describe in a more structured environment.

=== **POINTS TO REMEMBER** ===

- Make communication happen; Schedule time for it and set an agenda.

- Utilize the speaker/listener technique or another form of active listening.

- Set a time limit for the weekly check-in or other important discussions.

- If you do not cover all you had hoped during a check-in, either agree to extend the time or schedule another meeting.

- Practice active listening skills.

- Call a halt to the conversation if one or both of you is getting agitated or emotions are escalating.

- Agree that there is to be no yelling, no swearing, and no threats.

- Make sure both of you are clear on what you are agreeing to, what you are tabling for later, or what you have decided upon as an action plan.

For more resources, go to:

www.DrAnneMalec.com

CHAPTER THREE:

And the Evolution Continues

Change is constant throughout our lives and in our relationships. With the pace of technological change, cultural and family improvements in gender equality, and the common need for two career families, there is little doubt that the modern marriage needs to deal with a significant amount of flux. Changing job circumstances, relationship expectations, and life demands are to be expected, all requiring a willing acceptance and need for adaptation from both partners. And change does not have to be bad. Change very often brings with it novelty, which, as noted earlier, humans desire and relationships need.

On top of change caused by external forces, there are two types of change you should expect in your marriage: changes asked of you by your partner and changes your partner seeks for himself or herself in an effort to make life more interesting. We all continue to change and grow as we move through life, and so must our relationships. No one is a finished product.

Think back to when you were dating. You met this wonderful person. As your new love's personality revealed itself, each new layer was so interesting and exciting. You could not help but tell your friends and family how wonderful and fascinating this person was because he or she had so much going on! She was good at sailing and so cute and funny; he was brilliant at business and ran marathons. The fun of peeling back all these layers yielded surprises and revelations that made your new love intriguing.

Novelty—surprise—these things continue to interest and delight us throughout life, and they should not stop just because you are married. New activities and interests are one way to keep a relationship fresh. Sameness leads to boredom. None of us want to be boring or to be bored in our relationship. Each of us should help facilitate change and evolution in ourselves and our partners, as this enhances the relationship. So, why do we sometimes see change as threatening?

In part, change is perceived as a threat because when you marry someone you think you know that person fully. You see him or her as a best friend. You think you know what he is going to say or how she is going to act in certain situations. Such expectations establish a certain comfort level. Knowing someone well adds to our sense of safety and security, which human beings seek. There are fewer surprises; the consistency feels good. So, when your partner tells you, "I've decided I want to go back to school because my career as a real estate professional is increasingly unfulfilling," your notion of that person is suddenly challenged. You might think, "Wait, what's happening here? I thought I knew you. Why are you doing this? You say you're unfulfilled. Is it just your job? Are you bored with our life? Are you bored with me?"

But if partners realize change and personal growth have an upside, they can encourage it within their relationships. They will see it as enriching and far less threatening. If your partner thinks that he is going to be a happier person as a physician's assistant, is willing to commit to the additional education it requires, and you can make ends meet in the process, then you should try to support him in this endeavor.

Getting your spouse's buy-in will be much easier and more likely if the change is considered healthy and constructive for the relationship. If your partner is a little bored with himself and wants to change things up a little, or a lot, such as in his career, do not interpret this as your spouse saying, "I need a new partner." He is saying, "I need change, I need a new focus; I need a different goal in my life." It is normal and healthy to seek greater personal fulfillment. Within a relationship, this should be encouraged and supported.

To what extent do you need to get on board? When your partner tells you something like this, he wants you to be happy and excited and not minimize, dismiss, or poke holes in his ideas or plans. It can be hard not to react when the impact of the proposed change on your life is unpredictable. Even so, your relationship will benefit from putting your concerns aside and investing yourself in your partner's dream: learn about it, ask questions, and try to climb on board. You do not want your partner to feel like he or she is alone going down this path. And in sharing it, your partner is enlisting your help in reaching his or her goal. You are the most significant relationship in your partner's life, and your partner is seeking your encouragement and support. The need for support and understanding between partners does not mean honest discussion about your feelings comes off the table. It means that in your honest discussion, fears and anxieties need to be balanced with support, encouragement, and interest. Utilize your weekly check-in meetings to provide status updates or shifts in thinking about changes you and your partner have previously explored or proposed.

Again, communication is essential, whether you are the partner proposing the change or the partner hearing about it. When you sit down together, you need to be ready to listen, answer questions, and not be defensive or dismissive of concerns.

As the partner proposing the change, you owe your mate honest answers and thoughtful listening to his or her concerns. Your partner is unlikely to be as excited about the new idea as you are on first hearing about it. If you want your partner to be on board, think of what is important for you to communicate. If it is a major change in your life together, you should consider preparing a written document, whether that includes a budget, a business plan, or an education plan. Be prepared to address what you want to do and how you think it will impact your relationship and your family. The partner seeking change should never downplay the other partner's concerns about potential loss of income or increase in expenses. Spell it out, create projections, and consider the worst-case scenario, as plans rarely play out as hoped or expected.

What if a proposed change, new job, or business opportunity does not work? How much time will you give it to succeed? The partner hearing about a proposed change has the job of being the cheerleader *and* the reality checker. Life-changing goals or dreams are a tough thing to talk about; to frankly say, "I believe in you. I support you. I love you—but your dream cannot supersede every other dream or need of our family." Those communication skills we discussed in the preceding chapter are crucial here. Whatever the issues, talk through them patiently, thoughtfully, and with an open mind. Nobody wants to have a dream shot down, but both parties have to move forward with their eyes open.

Not all changes are career-related or follow someone's dream. Some change requests come from your partner and request changes in *you*. These can be the most difficult to manage individually and relationally because they require patience, openness, and extreme vulnerability.

"You must change the way you _____!" How can you fill in the blank from your relationship? We have probably all heard or said it at one point. Such a request can come when one party feels that there is an imbalance in the relationship. My experience reveals that these requests are hard to articulate effectively and even harder to hear. Asking a partner to change a behavior is seen by some as too confrontational, so one may try to make his or her feelings known through other means. Instead of making a clear request for change along with the reason for the request, partners may drop hints: verbally, behaviorally, or passive-aggressively. If this is you, challenge yourself to communicate respectfully to your partner about what change you are seeking and why it means so much to you. If need be, put it on your weekly meeting agenda.

A spouse may seek change from a partner when feeling that he or she is giving too much and not getting enough in return or feels the relationship lacks balance in some other way. Social scientists use "equity theory" to describe this situation.[11] Equity theory proposes that individuals who perceive themselves as either under-rewarded or over-rewarded in a relationship will experience distress; that distress leads to an effort to restore equity within the relationship. The theory also considers whether the distribution of resources is fair to both partners, with fairness determined by the ratios of contributions and benefits for both parties in the relationship.

What do I bring to this relationship? Is my partner bringing something of equal value? These types of questions are frequently asked of ourselves when dating; we also tend to choose potential mates around this concept of equity. We tend to feel that the other should bring an equivalent amount to the relationship table, in looks, education, success, potential, experience, and so on. Whether or not we measure a partner's value this directly, to be deemed attractive a potential mate needs to at least match or ideally exceed our view of what we bring. This is naturally subjective and tends to fluctuate over time.

Couples in relationships constantly, if only subconsciously, make this "is it fair" calculation, especially as it relates to income, the division of household tasks, and child-care responsibilities. The partner who feels that the relationship is unbalanced, who feels "I am putting in significantly more than he is or she is," needs to muster the courage to talk to his or her partner about it. Do not count on your partner being able to read your mind (see ineffective communication strategies in the previous chapter). As difficult and uncomfortable as this discussion may be, the poor alternative is expressing your feelings in an unproductive way, often when you are angry, frustrated, or feeling overwhelmed with annoyance. Focus on how you feel in the bothersome situation and what you need to make it right. Then ask your partner for what you need: "Coming home from work and having to cook five nights a week is exhausting. I need help." Or, "I can't handle paying all the bills and managing the investment accounts every month. It's too much of a burden for me. I need to share some of this with you." Or, "I can't always be the main contact with the child-care providers and the kids' school—I need you to participate more."

When a spouse asks for a change in behavior, it can sometimes feel like he or she is trying to control you or insult your go-to way of being. It can be hard to hear. But if you consider that your partner is doing it to share a frustration because he or she does not want it to be a continuing problem, it is easier to see the change request as a potential benefit for your relationship. Your partner is trying to stay connected and close to you, so you should listen to what he or she has to say. The subtext of your partner's request is, "This situation bothers me," or "I'm feeling like you expect me to do a lot more than you expect of yourself." Your partner is expressing discontent or worse—resentment—and sharing it with you, and it is a good thing that he or she is being open about it because unaddressed resentment in a marriage is toxic. If your partner tries to tell you that he or she is feeling that things are out of balance in your relationship, and you dismiss the feelings as criticism or respond defensively, your partner may feel like he or she cannot talk to you. Consequently, your partner might stop opening up to you altogether. When conversation stops, resentment starts. That is an outcome you want to avoid if your goal is to sustain a happy, healthy marriage.

That being said, requests for change in your partner's behavior are only effective in moderation. You have heard it before, but it is true: you must pick your battles. A highly respected marriage researcher, John Gottman, recommends that spouses work to keep a 5:1 ratio of positive/negative interactions.[12] I second his guidance. If you feel a need to ask your partner to change, make sure you make a point of communicating the things you love about your partner and that he or she does right!

If you find that much of your partner's behavior is bothersome to you, even after you read chapter 4 of this book, it might be time to talk to a mental health professional. Some habits or behaviors that worked well when you were single might not transition well to married life. The goal is to figure out a way to live together amicably, romantically, and pragmatically. Compromise is a requirement. Whether the issue is related to the temperature in your home, grocery store shopping habits, weekend schedules, or something else, neither one of you is wrong; you just have different preferences. You are going to need to talk about this and figure out the best way forward.

Sometimes requests for change are related to a personality trait or attitude and not a specific behavior. A common topic in my practice is one spouse asking another to change an attitude. Usually, it involves a partner feeling the other is too negative or cynical. With requests like this that are abstract and very much a part of a personality structure, partners can become understandably defensive. The defensiveness is often a reaction to feeling hurt and scared by the request. Let's face it: knowing there is a part of us that our partners do not like feels like a threat to our relationship. For the partner asking for the change, it is important that you frame your request delicately and be considerate about the timing. Requests of this type made in the midst of an argument will not go well. Set yourself up to succeed: how you articulate your request matters a great deal in this situation, and it might help to practice beforehand what you plan to say. Be mindful of the need for a respectful tone of voice, a gentle introduction of the topic, and empathy for your partner's feelings. For example: "You know I love how intelligent, thoughtful, and funny you are. But sometimes I think when you are trying to be pragmatic and realistic, you come across as overly pessimistic or cynical. I do not think you are as negative as you sometimes sound. It would mean a lot to me if you would try to moderate some of your comments."

Can negative attitudes be altered? Can a glass half-empty partner become a glass half-full partner? With steady effort and thoughtfulness, it is possible to change how you think and react. It is hard to change—but to achieve harmony in some areas, including our intimate relationships, we have to be willing to try. Stubbornness is often held up as a point of pride; but, in a relationship, all it means is that you are proudly inflexible. Although changing habits and thoughts may be difficult, it is possible. It means building new relationship muscles, thinking before reflexively speaking or acting, and not losing sight of the value your partner brings to your life. Rejecting your partner's request for change has a subtext that says, "I don't care. That's just who I am, and I'll live with the consequences if you don't like it." If this sounds like you, you might find it worthwhile to think about what keeps you from being willing to consider your partner's request for change. What relationship benefits do you see to being negative or pessimistic?

There are points in every relationship when one partner has said to the other, "You do this thing that bugs the heck out of me. Please, can you stop it?" It is not an attack on you—your spouse is saying "I want to keep you close. I want to keep this good. I want to continue to love you, so please hear me when I ask you to look at this thing that you're doing." It is probably fair to say that none of us look forward to hearing what our partners think we need to change. However, ignoring respectful pleas or denying requests for change will create frustration and will lead your partner to feel unheard, disrespected, and angry. Feelings of anger run the risk of becoming resentment and could motivate a partner to demand changes more often, hoping to find *something* that you are willing to change and that shows you care. Most likely, a request for change that gets ignored will continue to simmer in the background and become a bigger problem later. It will serve your marriage well if you are both open to hearing a partner's request for change and exhibit a willingness to address the issue. To stand the best chance of being heard when making a request, be as specific and respectful as possible.

What behaviors are fair to ask your partner to change?

- Sloppiness

- Overspending

- Inequities in the household division of child care, cooking, cleaning, yard work, laundry, and managing finances.

- A lack of interest in sexual intimacy (see chapter 7).

- Changing his or her resistance to spontaneity.

- Paying more attention to his or her health.

- Paying attention to his or her intake of intoxicating or harmful substances.

- Seeking help for addictions.

- Moderating overwhelming pessimism/negativity.

- Limiting the accumulation of stuff (whether you call it collecting or hoarding depends on your point of view).

I cannot stress enough that the key here is the moderation in requests and the importance of the ratio of positive to negative comments. No one likes to feel *so* imperfect or that a partner does not think he or she is good enough. Your partner is a completely different person than you are, with a different background, perspective, opinions, likes, dislikes, and bad habits. All of us have them. Accept the ones you can and respectfully ask your partner to change some others. But also be open to similar requests for yourself.

How do you make a request for change respectful? Invite the other to the conversation. Put it on the agenda. It is important to state how you feel about what the other is doing. Be as specific as possible about what behavior bothers you, how it makes you feel, and what your partner can do to change. For example, "I'm concerned that we are consuming a bottle of wine every night. I have half a glass, and you finish the bottle." It could be, "I am fearful that you are going to get sick. Heart disease runs in your family, and you're not exercising. It would mean a lot to me if you would pay more attention to your health."

As the partner being asked to change, listen, paraphrase, ask for clarification if needed, and consider the request. Defensiveness or reflexively rejecting what your partner has to say kills the discussion. Shutting down the discussion might feel like the right thing in the moment, but it sends the wrong message to your partner and will make him or her less likely to communicate with you in the future. You can win the battle but lose the war. Use the communication guidelines from the previous chapter, and try using the speaker/listener technique if you find you or your partner becoming emotionally reactive.

There may be some requests for change that you feel cross the line of emotional, sexual, or physical safety. You may feel that your partner is asking too much of you or asking you to engage in behaviors that make you feel uncomfortable. If this occurs, try talking with your partner about why it makes you uncomfortable, and see if you might find a compromise. If you do not feel safe talking about these issues with your partner, it may be time to consult with a mental health professional who can provide an additional perspective and insight.

STUFF HAPPENS: Life throws all kinds of changes at us that affect our relationships and may be out of our control. Continue to problem-solve and communicate frequently about the best ways to tackle and manage these life events.

Some common life-changing events include:

- Change of career.
- Extended family members needing help.
- A desire to return to school for more education.
- A high-earning partner/parent decides to become a stay-at-home parent.
- A partner develops depression, anxiety, or seems angry all the time.
- Your partner no longer seems interested in parenting.
- A partner loses his or her job.
- Your spouse gets a debilitating illness, which means he or she cannot work and requires home-based care.
- Your spouse gets fired. Maybe more than once.
- Your spouse makes bad investment choices and wipes out much of your retirement savings.
- A partner is offered a job transfer in a different city.
- Your parents need to move in with you because they did not properly plan for their retirement.

- You have a child who has learning, emotional, or developmental difficulties.

The conundrum is that the harder things are to talk about, the more you must talk about them. Without healthy dialogue and the safe conversational space to share your thoughts and feelings, the issue will eventually get presented in the midst of a fight, through passive-aggressive behavior, or through the explosive release of built-up resentment. When change is inevitable, we owe each other the respect that comes with knowing we are in this together.

In this discussion of change, what needs to remain constant and unchanging? Mutual respect and a safe space for conversation top the list. You also need a willingness to accept that a lot of what partners disagree about may not require complete resolution to live harmoniously—and that is okay. Hardly anything in life is black and white; how boring life would be if it were. The important thing is that you talk about it, hear your partner's concerns, try to find middle ground, and brainstorm solutions together. This is mutual respect in action.

In summary, learn not to fear change in your life or your relationship. Change does not have to be threatening, and it will happen. The result can and often does enhance relationships. Change is evolution and personal growth. Viewed in this light, you want your partner to change, and you should be changing too!

===== POINTS TO REMEMBER =====

- Change is an inevitable part of life—and without it, we would not grow and would become increasingly bored and boring.

- Your spouse may have a dream or game plan that would mean significant changes for you both. When it comes up, try not to react with reflexive negativity, but listen thoughtfully, and consider what he or she is saying.

- It is normal in the course of a relationship that you and your partner will find some habits or customary behaviors of the other off-putting. It is perfectly okay to express this and ask for change as long as you do not overdo these requests. Make your request in a respectful and caring way.

- If your partner asks you to change something that irritates him or her, do not take it as an insult or an attempt to control you.

- Refusing to hear your partner's request for change feels disrespectful and dismissive. These ignored requests can frequently lead to anger and resentment.

For more resources, go to:
www.DrAnneMalec.com

CHAPTER FOUR:

What You Need to Bring

Remember when you were a kid and going to a sleepover or a field trip or off to camp? You usually received a list of things that you needed to bring with you to cover contingencies. You probably did not receive a list when you committed to a romantic relationship (however, it is funny to imagine the different reactions to the exchanging of such lists!). But there are a number of responsibilities that you need to cover to maintain a healthy and happy long-term relationship. This chapter discusses important things you need to create a successful relationship. Too often, one's expectations are about what a partner should do for you without equal thought and consideration given to your partner's needs. Make a commitment to bring the following important elements to your relationship.

WHAT TO BRING TO YOUR PARTNER:

Remain Kind, Thoughtful, and Generous.

Relationships require us to give and not just to take, to be generous when we may feel selfish, and to be considerate of the other when we want it to be our turn. Part of being an "us" is being willing at times to put your personal needs second. You will never regret treating your partner with kindness, but you will regret treating your partner with disdain. Yes, we all have stresses and anxieties. We all have bad days and bad moods. There will be times when you act self-centered and even a little selfish. But in the big picture, you have to give as much or more than you receive.

All of us should be willing to give our partners a pass and cut him or her some slack if we know that he or she is under a lot of stress or feeling tension from issues outside of the relationship. There are times in each of our lives when stress outside our marriage will cause friction inside the marriage. If your partner occasionally acts like a jerk, consider what stressors or competing time demands he or she is facing outside of the relationship. Remember, it is not always about you. Do not assume it is and make the situation even more stressful for your partner. Often a partner's current unpleasantness is not a reflection of how he or she feels about you, nor is it a reflection of your partner's true character. This, too, shall pass.

Sometimes our partners need our sympathy and support—they need us to walk with them as they process feelings of hurt or disappointment. The gift our partners receive in such a situation is the knowledge that they are not alone. They do not want to hear a platitude such as, "You've got nothing to worry about." If they felt they had nothing to worry about, they would not be worried. Your partner needs you to listen to his or her struggles and to understand why he or she is sad, disappointed, or troubled. Before you can conquer an obstacle together, you need first to empathize with what your partner is feeling. You need to be with your partner in his or her moment of pain or struggle, without judgment, without minimization, by *being present*.

Let your partner hear your support and know that you have his or her back. Even if you are confident that the big picture may be more nuanced than what you are hearing, remember that you are on your spouse's team. Your partner comes to you for love and support. Give it freely, and save the brainstorming for another time. Patient supportiveness can be hard for some people, especially for the successful take-charge types whose professional success may be due to instinctively jumping right in to start "fixing" whatever appears broken. Empathy goes a long way, as does a loving question, like, "How are you doing? You seem kind of stressed. Can I help?" Very often, this approach can diffuse the situation and give your partner a chance to vent. It reminds your partner that you are on his or her team.

Actively Notice and Admire Your Partner.

It is interesting how, when we live with someone, it can become hard to see him or her clearly after a while. As we get used to situations and the people around us, we can too easily forget what initially attracted us. It is similar to when you buy a new car or a new home. Remember how much you loved it and obsessed over it? You could not wait to drive it, could not wait to move into your new home and show it off to your friends and family. Six months later, it is just a way to get from one place to another or rest your head. This is normal human behavior. After a while, people tend to stop noticing what initially excited them. We habituate to even the very best things in life—so be aware of this danger.

After living with a partner for years, we can lose focus on the many wonderful things he or she does and can become annoyed with things a partner does not do or does less well. If you are looking for something negative, you usually are going to find it. It is good to recall frequently why you fell in love with your partner.

Keep in touch with and keep your eye on those loveable, adorable traits that initially drew you in. Especially when you are struggling or when the not-so-good traits are frustrating, consider, "What attracted me at first?"

Making a gratitude list can be very helpful in maintaining a positive perspective (I do it while sitting in Chicago's traffic to help manage my commute annoyance). List what is good in your relationship and what your partner brings to your life and, from time to time, share it with your partner. That sharing requires making yourself vulnerable, and it just might make him or her blush. No one ever tires of receiving compliments from a spouse. Make it a priority to notice the small healthy changes that your partner makes, offer encouragement and support, point out his or her strengths and choose to see the best in him or her. Look your partner in the eye when you talk to him or her and when he or she is talking to you. Take the time to notice your partner: things like, "Wow, he looks nice in blue," or "She always looks great whenever she leaves the house."

Being married does not mean that your partner no longer needs to hear that you think he or she is cute, attractive, sexy, hot, and so on. Do not neglect saying so, or you run the risk of your partner believing you no longer think this way. If you have trouble finding things to admire or for which to be grateful, you need to change your glasses, figuratively speaking. If this is how you truly feel, that there is nothing to like or admire about your mate, it shows. Your spouse will feel it, and it is detrimental to your relationship. Based upon my clinical observation, what is more common than a true lack of admiration is a lack of communicating that admiration.

Take Responsibility for Expressing Appreciation and Gratitude.

This is a common issue in distressed relationships: a perceived lack of appreciation or gratitude for what the other brings to the relationship. No person I have encountered clinically has ever expressed boredom with hearing what a romantic partner appreciates about him or her. Create reminders if you must! (My stepson and stepdaughter-in-law have typed the words "Love him" and "Love her" in their cell phones next to each other's names, as a constant reminder of their mutual affection.) Make it a practice to tell your partner what you appreciate about him or her at least once a day. Share how thankful you are that he or she took out the trash, planted the garden, shoveled the snow, walked the dog, arranged for the babysitter, made a delicious dinner, or acted as the in-house tech person. You get my point.

Expressions of gratitude for daily efforts go a lot further than birthday gifts or anniversary cards in letting your partner feel like you appreciate all that he or she does. Partners will sometimes say, "Why would I have to thank him when what he is doing also benefits him?" The answer is because it is an expression of love, and none of us like to feel taken for granted.

I frequently hear clients say how much they want and need to receive a partner's appreciation for the income he or she brings to the family. A partner needs to hear that his or her spouse appreciates all the hard work and effort put toward earning an income. Spouses frequently seek validation at home because he or she is not hearing it at the office. The need for appreciation and validation is an often overlooked aspect of relationships. It can be addressed simply by saying to your partner, "I know you're working very hard, and I'm very thankful for it because you bring a lot to our family." This always feels good to hear.

Do not be stingy about expressing your gratitude. A simple, heartfelt "thank you" goes a long way—add in a hug and a kiss for the trifecta.

Be Considerate, Respectful, and Polite.
Actions that fall under this category include:

- Asking your partner if he or she needs anything from the kitchen if you are heading that way.

- Letting your partner sleep in while you get up with the kids.

- Looking to see what needs to be done without waiting to be asked.

- Not committing to a social engagement without first checking with your partner.

- Developing the habit of communicating if you are going to be late getting home.

- Remembering that the two of you share an account and not making large withdrawals without telling the other about it.

- Giving your partner privacy.

- Giving your partner time and space for self-care and acknowledging when you need time for yourself without growing resentful or needy.

- Shutting the bathroom door as well as knocking first.

- Recognizing that just because you turned on the television, it does not mean you own the remote for the day.

All of us know to be respectful of others, but it is even more important that you show good manners to your partner. Some suggestions:

- Do not use sarcasm—it is often just another form of expressed anger.

- Do not insult or call your partner names—even if you think it is only a joke (especially about specific body parts).

- Always watch your tone of voice, and do not shout from a different room.

- Do not yell. Do. Not. Yell. Ever.

There is no room for yelling in a marriage. It will never get you what you want, unless you want an angry partner. When someone yells, the blood pressure of all those within earshot goes up. Perhaps you have thought, "I have to yell. It's the only way that he hears me," or, "I've already said it five other times, so now I have to yell for her to take me seriously." When you yell, your partner gets upset and agitated to the point that whatever point you were trying to make will be completely lost, and all that he or she hears is your anger and disrespectful tone. One yelling partner can rather easily become two yelling partners. Then you are off to the races, and what could have been a simple exchange has escalated into a major negative interaction.

WHAT TO BRING TO YOUR RELATIONSHIP:

Prioritize Your Intimate Relationship.

In the course of my work, I frequently suggest to couples that they sit and talk to each other for ten minutes per day. Not everyone follows through with my suggestion, which indicates to me that if it is too hard to find ten minutes for a spouse, your marriage is not a priority to you. Your relationship will atrophy, just like an unused muscle. Sometimes couples even have trouble finding the time to share a hug and kiss upon arrivals and departures. How much time is too much to keep your relationship strong and loving? How many less consequential things take up 30 seconds of your day? Refocus, reprioritize, and strengthen your bond.

The fact is that you and your children will suffer if you do not focus on the couple relationship. Even if life events intervene and you miss a week or two of making time for each other, do not let it become a habit. It is so, so important to carve out couple time, to find the time to say, "Our relationship is the most important thing in our lives." A nonfunctioning relationship will have a negative impact on every other aspect of your life. Make sure your weekends do not become overly scheduled with activities that you wind up with no "us" time. Focus on creating the time and space in which you two come first for each other.

Willingly Share Responsibility.
In modern relationships, it is fair to expect to share equal responsibility for raising your children, providing financial support, and completing household tasks. Remember, just because your parents split the work a specific way does not mean that your relationship needs to function the same way. Determine what you consider to be a fair sharing of responsibility, and always be willing to readjust as required by life's changes.

Create New Traditions.
Part of prioritizing your relationship means prioritizing the new over the old. When you marry, you make a commitment to another person and create a new family. This new family will have

its boundaries, values, and traditions. The two of you may decide to do things differently than both of your birth families in where you take vacations, how you spend money, who provides child care, and where your children go to school. Be mindful of not letting your birth families become too influential as you create your new family.

Put Limits on Your Use of Technology When Together.

As noted in chapter 1, technology can have a negative impact on intimate relationships. No one wants to feel that his or her partner needs to look for entertainment elsewhere when spending time together. And that is what it looks like when you pick up your cell phone during an evening out. Prioritizing your relationship and showing appreciation for your partner requires a commitment on your part to be fully present and engaged when you are together. Checking your email, playing apps, and texting other people needs to be put on hold now and then and especially during daily check-ins or weekly meetings. You need to show your partner that you care enough to give him or her your full attention.

Be Committed and Faithful in Your Relationship.

Finding others attractive is normal and natural. As human beings, we are attracted to pretty, new, shiny things. But marriage is a commitment to your partner that you will not act on feelings of attraction toward other people. Monogamous commitment is a choice. You need your choice to be: "I'm faithful to my partner every day, even when I may be angry or hurt or feeling distant." Your relationship is your most valuable asset. Being unfaithful *always* screws things up, quite often irretrievably. It is harder to repair broken trust after infidelity than it is to build it in the first place. Avoid the pull of being unfaithful and instead use any feelings you may have in that direction as motivation to access and discuss what may be missing in your marriage.

Sometimes it is helpful to view marriage as a bank account, an account into which we make deposits every day. Relationship deposits are a result of:

- treating your partner respectfully,

- being interested in your partner,

- prioritizing your partner and relationship,

- giving affection,

- being considerate and supportive,

- listening well, and

- a myriad of other efforts made in service to your relationship.

Like a good retirement account, steady deposits lead to healthy returns.

BRING YOUR BEST SELF.

Take Care of Yourself.

When you met your partner, you were physically attracted to each other—or your relationship would not have gotten off the ground. As people age over the length of a marriage, time takes its toll. Some may feel that external appearances should not matter as much as they did initially because your partner is supposed to love you for what is on the inside. Your partner should love your inner qualities, but relying exclusively on this belief can lead to bad habits such as not exercising, neglecting your appearance, and gaining weight. Getting married does not give you a free pass to stop putting care into your appearance and physical health.

While all of us want our partners to love what is on the inside, the outside matters, too. It is human to desire an attractive partner and to want others to view us as having an attractive partner. How each of you looks reflects upon the other. I acknowledge that what is deemed attractive varies to some degree, and this is not an argument for superficiality. Rather, it is a suggestion that you discover what you and your partner find attractive, and make an effort to nurture the aspects that are within your control.

If you want to keep attraction alive and keep intimacy and sexual desire thriving, it makes sense to continue to take care of yourself. Yes, it is tough, particularly as you age, but it should be a priority. Why? Partners can become resentful and angry when their spouses stop trying. Desire may lessen, and the spouse who is out of shape may avoid sex because he or she does not feel attractive. The negative effects for both partners puts additional strain on the relationship. Do not save your best looks and grooming for the office; put forth the same effort at home! Who are you trying to impress if not the person who means the most to you? (There is great irony in the common behavior of paying increased attention to appearance when newly divorced or separated and preparing to enter the dating market.)

Bring Emotional Health to Your Marriage.
If you suffer from depression or anxiety, take the initiative and seek help. If your partner says he or she thinks you may have a problem with drinking, instead of becoming defensive, consider whether it might be true. In my clinical observation, it is rare for a partner to admit to problem-drinking until confronted with how much he or she is actually consuming. Unfortunately, in our culture, alcoholism is a very common problem. If your partner sees a change in you and becomes concerned, but you do not want

to hear it, fight your resistance to deny—and listen. The same goes for depression, stress, and anxiety. Instead of seeing this comment as judgment, try to see it as an expression of love and concern. Nine times out of ten, in my experience, spouses do not raise these issues to be hurtful but because they are worried. Bring a willingness to listen and keep your defensiveness in check.

Be Willing to Change Your Bad Habits.

Bad habits might include smoking, drinking, recreational drug use, or even just bad table manners. Whatever it is, make sure it does not turn into a wedge issue or a turn-off for your partner. Pay extra attention to curbing those habits that your partner has requested that you change. If you repeatedly resist your partner's requests for change, he or she may stop asking. This is not a sign the problem has dissipated, it might have just morphed into resentment. Go ahead and ask your partner for support in changing your bad habits and maintaining a healthier lifestyle.

COMMUNICATION SKILLS YOU NEED TO BRING:

Commit to Being Honest with Your Partner.

Honesty matters in ways large and small. Your spouse needs to be able to believe what you say and vice versa. Dishonesty creates unease in a relationship that can fester like a wound. Withholding important information is dishonest; it is lying by omission. Some justify lying by believing the truth would only upset one's partner. The truth may hurt your partner, but that does not justify dishonesty. The problem with being untruthful is that if your partner finds out about it, which partners usually do, you create a situation where he or she will begin to doubt everything you say.

It is a slippery slope that leads to an erosion in trust and reliability, so avoid it whenever possible.

Trust Your Partner's Commitment to You.

Trust that your partner always has your best interests in mind; that even though he or she may be angry or stressed, it might not have anything to do with you. Trust that if your partner does have a problem with you, he or she will tell you. If your partner becomes distracted by a life event requiring full focus and attention, such as a work, family, or health issue, trust that it is a temporary situation and part of the ebb and flow of a long-term relationship. Do not automatically view it as an act of selfishness or a rejection of "us." It is okay to discuss concerns or insecurities with your partner, but when he or she reassures you and expresses his or her commitment, it is your responsibility to believe your partner.

Bring Your Vulnerability.

Vulnerability is a vital component of healthy couple communication. Trusting that you can show your spouse the parts of yourself that embarrass or shame you, the parts that you may have kept hidden from others, or of which you are not proud allows your partner to know the real you. Vulnerability is trusting that you can share who you are and that your partner will accept you without judgment. While we hope for complete acceptance, we cannot know for sure if we will receive it, so being vulnerable with another person is an emotional risk.

I experienced vulnerability in my marriage by sharing with my husband my struggle since childhood with stuttering. For the first few decades of my life, my stutter brought me great shame and embarrassment. I saw it as my personal handicap that would strike when I most needed to speak clearly. I tried to hide it as best

I could. I would like to say that it is no longer an issue for me, but in truth, from time to time it still happens and continues to embarrass me. As I see in my work, childhood insecurities often last into adulthood.

As I began to feel secure in our relationship, I eventually shared with my husband my struggle. I spoke of the outsized role it played in my life, my constant vigilance to hide it, and the effect on my self-image. Sharing these deep insecurities was incredibly freeing for me, as it led to greater self-acceptance and increased compassion for the young girl I once was. It helped me feel closer to my husband because vulnerability fosters intimacy and connection. When we are vulnerable with those to whom we are closest, it makes it easier to be vulnerable with others. It indeed can be life changing.

Vulnerability is a two-way street: just as we bring it to our partners and hope for emotional safety, we also need to provide the same safety for them. When we open ourselves up to love, we also open ourselves to the possibility of hurt, of pain. But the good outweighs the bad, so go ahead and share your vulnerability, because you want your partner to share his or hers, too. One-sided vulnerability may lead to no vulnerability, which can eventually deprive a relationship of intimacy.

Be Willing to Listen.

Part of listening means remembering what your partner says. Why? Because it is the best way to show your partner that you are listening and that what they say is important. Looking directly at your partner when you communicate will increase your odds of remembering. Another way to pay attention and remember your partner's requests or concerns is to make sure your 20-minute daily check-in is screen-free time.

Be willing to listen even when you disagree or when you have heard the story before. Listen even when you are not following the story or your partner is going off on a tangent. Listen even when you think your partner is wrong. You have a responsibility to make a real effort to listen respectfully and trust your partner will do the same for you. Listening is part of the glue that holds relationships together.

Be Willing to Talk.

Communication is mandatory. You may be stoic, or you might feel like you do not have a lot to say, but your partner wants to— needs to—hear from you. Being silent does not mean you can avoid problems, because they still exist even when you do not talk about them. Unaddressed problems often fester, growing more complicated with time. The longer an issue goes unaddressed, the lower the likelihood of it ever being resolved.

It is not unusual for one partner to enjoy talking more than the other. There is nothing wrong with this. However, even if you do not feel a strong need to talk, be mindful that it is part of the bargain of marriage. You are responsible for contributing to the lifetime of conversations. Ask about your partner's day, his or her favorite sports team, family, work project, the book he or she is reading, or current events. Conversation is a way to show you are interested in your partner. It is *very* important.

Separate careers keep many of us apart from our mates for so many hours each day that it is important to ask about, follow up with, and to connect with them about current work issues or complications. Knowing that your partner is aware of your work anxieties and concerns goes a long way to fostering connection. Make it a habit to check in via phone, text, or email midway through your day. Who does not appreciate reading a love text just after a tough meeting?

Those partners with school-age children habitually ask their children about school, what they did, what they learned, who they sat next to during lunch, and so on. Your partner needs that same level of attention and interest from you. Although circumstances on a given day may mean you give less time to your partner than your children, your spouse should never be made to feel that he or she is less important than your children. Remember, your partner was number one before kids and most likely enjoyed that ranking.

Do Not Swing at Pitches in the Dirt.

There are going to be times when your partner takes an easy jab that pokes you in a soft spot and upsets you. Do not rise to the bait. Take a breath, think before you speak, and maybe decide not to speak at all. It only takes one person to stop an argument from happening. It should go without saying that you should try to avoid taking cheap shots; you almost always feel worse after the fact. When you feel the need to make a point to your spouse, choose the issues that are of core importance to you and make your discussions around them constructive.

Bickering wastes time. For many couples, it turns into a nasty habit. The real issue behind bickering is winning. However, there is no winner with chronic bickering. You cannot have a winner-take-all mindset in a loving, long-term marriage, because if someone has to win, then someone else has to lose. Losing feels lousy and affects both partners negatively, even the "winner." Be aware that if this has become habitual in your relationship, it is probably masking an underlying issue that needs attention.

Agree Not to Fight Via Text Message.

With the frequency of communication via text message ever increasing, arguing via text is now a common means of conflict. Work to avoid this habit. It is too easy to send a hurtful text message mindlessly. And it is very risky to entrust your relationship to the quite-often abbreviated and auto-corrected word. Find a time to discuss an issue in person, or if it is time sensitive, use email instead of text messaging. Email gives you the opportunity to think and read through what you are saying. Try to read the message from your partner's perspective. Is there something that your partner can take the wrong way? Find another way to word what you want to say in a more direct and considerate manner. And, it never hurts to let a harsh message sit in your draft folder for an hour or two, and reread and soften it when emotions have decreased.

Be Willing to Forgive and to Seek Forgiveness.

This can be a tough one, depending on the perceived infraction, calling on each of you to be vulnerable in a time of emotional pain. But I believe the responsibility to forgive should be included in wedding vows because every relationship requires it. Failure to forgive is dangerous. It can make you physically sick, thanks to the toxic energy that comes from keeping a running tally of hurts, disappointments, and the shortcomings of your partner. Be especially wary of holding onto a grudge for an infraction your partner is not even aware of committing. If you are upset at something your partner did, tell him or her. Waiting for your partner to guess what has upset you sets a harmful precedent and makes it more likely the hurt will morph into resentment for both of you.

Stubbornness is not a virtue in your relationship. There is nothing gained and a lot lost by refusing to apologize. Vulnerability plays a significant role in asking for forgiveness, because in taking responsibility for our actions, we need to trust that our partners will forgive without shaming us. Shaming your partner will destroy the possibility of vulnerability. What does shaming look like in a relationship? Shaming is:

- Pointing out a partner's weaknesses or telling outsiders about them.

- Using past honesty as an emotional weapon.

- Humiliating your partner when he or she makes a mistake.

- Laughing at your partner's expense.

- Expressing derision in a moment of vulnerability.

You can forgive without waiting for your partner to ask you for forgiveness. Forgive of your own free will simply because it feels good. It can be emotionally freeing to *think* something along the lines of, "I am ruminating on this thing that you said or did, and I'm resentful about it. It is taking up too much space for me in in my heart and my head. Even though I think you were a total jerk, and you didn't apologize, I'm going to let it go because it's better for my life, and it's better for our marriage." You can verbalize this to your partner with a simple "I forgive you." Even if you still think he or she was a "total jerk," I suggest you skip that part and focus on what he or she could do better next time.

Keeping an upset to yourself out of fear of having a difficult discussion or confrontation with your partner does not usually work. Fear and avoidance of a confrontation usually leads to acting out your feelings through passive-aggressive behavior, a supremely ineffective method of communicating your feelings. Instead, choose to have the conversation. Find a time and place that you can discuss how the actions or words made you feel. Your partner may apologize or not, but at least you will have made your partner aware of how his or her actions affected you.

HONOR YOUR PARTNER AS A SEPARATE INDIVIDUAL:

Encourage Your Partner's Autonomy and Independence.

By this, I mean that there is no need to spend every moment together. We all need time away for self-care, reflection, processing, emotional recharging, or maybe just room *not* to talk. You cannot expect your partner to spend every nonworking free moment with you, nor do you need to spend it with your partner. We all need marriage-friendly extracurricular activities. It keeps you and your spouse interesting to yourselves and one another.

Your partner should also be allowed some freedom in personal decision-making, such as buying a new car or accepting a new job. There should be consultations with you, of course, but there also needs to be some autonomy for each of you to make the decisions that are best for you within the context of your family's interests. You do not have to understand why your partner wants to do everything that he or she does, and you should not judge him or her for it. The critical part is that individual decisions are being made in conjunction with the family's needs.

See Your Spouse as Competent.

You probably chose for your partner someone with an IQ similar to yours. That means your partner is equally capable of making decisions, whether about child rearing, how to load the dishwasher, or the route to take downtown. This is an issue that comes up a lot in therapy: a spouse who sees doing something differently as doing something wrong. But you did not marry your mate to parent them; you married an equal partner. With equality comes the expectation that your partner can make decisions on his or her own—without your input, assistance, help, or perspective.

Constantly correcting behavior gets old very quickly to the person being corrected; it is a total turn-off. And people who nag do not tend to enjoy their position in the dynamic either. Attempts at "correcting" are usually more about getting your partner to do it your way, so let it go or find a way to rectify the troubling situation yourself. Criticisms and corrections can feel particularly jarring for a spouse who is professionally very successful and comes home to face a litany of his or her shortcomings and failures. "You did this wrong. You forgot this. You overlooked that." This situation is dangerous in a marriage because it sets the stage for the "corrected" partner to not want to come home. It can feel not only very parental but trigger the least favorite memories of the child-parent relationship.

I have yet to meet someone who finds it helpful to be constantly corrected by his or her partner. If you are frequently criticizing or correcting your spouse, you should know it is not only harmful to your relationship but also completely ineffective as a motivator. Ask for what you need, let your partner do it his or her way, and treat your partner like the competent adult you married.

Cherish Your Differences.

Rarely are people attracted to someone who shares the same exact ideology or beliefs. Human beings crave complementarity in romantic partners, often to better themselves. For example, someone who is very social might choose a mate who is more introverted because this balances his or her need to be around other people while also prioritizing quiet time. Years later, the more outgoing partner may become frustrated with the introverted partner's tendency to always prefer a night in over going out with friends. Just as it would feel unfair to you if your partner grew tired of some of your innate and more "fixed" traits, it also feels unfair to him or her. This potential area of conflict calls for a work-around and a problem-solving strategy. Try to remember why you found this now-annoying quirk attractive in the beginning and change your glasses, figuratively speaking.

People have opposing ideas about many things, and that is okay. When you constantly resist your partner's opinions, feelings, and thoughts by being dismissive or belittling, it creates resent-ment. Remember, there is more than one way to load a dishwasher.

BRING YOUR WILLINGNESS TO MANAGE A LONG-TERM RELATIONSHIP.

Be Mindful to Control Your Impulses.

If you have a short fuse, are impatient, or easy to anger, recognize that this is a harmful characteristic that needs attention. Otherwise, it could lead to impaired marital communication. If a partner thinks that every discussion leads to a fight, he or she may back away from talking. If *you* have the short fuse, it is not your partner's fault that you lose your temper because he or she says something that bothers you. All of us are responsible for our actions and reactions. You may benefit from self-coaching to moderate your reactions if you tend to be sarcastic or reflexively defensive or dismissive. If a past interaction with your spouse spun out of control, spend time thinking about how you could have handled your side of things better.

Be Mindful of Your Complaining.

It is important to self-monitor how frequently you express negative statements to your partner. Even insignificant micro complaints about your partner add up. Statements such as "You're doing it wrong—it's better if you do it this way" or "Why would you do that?" or "I really wish you would …" have a cumulative effect. Ask yourself, *would I have acted this way in the first month of our relationship?* The answer is, probably not. What your partner hears is criticism, and everyone hates criticism. This bears repeating: Everyone hates criticism.

Complaints are allowed, of course, just be mindful of their frequency, and make sure you counter them with positive statements (remember the 5:1 ratio from chapter 3). When you have a complaint, communicate it very respectfully and specifically: "Could you please put your dirty clothes in the hamper?" as opposed to "You're such a slob!" Taking a shot at your spouse's habits quite often begets being on the receiving end of the same treatment. If you take this course, be ready to accept some complaints and corrections yourself.

Work on Patience and Tolerance Daily.

Being exposed to your partner's habits day after day, year after year can trigger feelings of annoyance in the most patient of partners. This is true even of habits that are not overtly "wrong." For example, I am sensitive to sound. I am annoyed by what I consider to be unnecessary noise (I think it might be genetic). When my husband is doing something completely normal and necessary—like chewing, finding something in the tool cabinet, or listening to music—and it is loud, I have to do deep breathing so that I do not react. In turn, my husband has an issue with what he considers clutter (he struggles to understand my reluctance to throw away slightly used paper towels, for example) and probably does his version of deep breathing to deal with that.

Do what you can to not react, to not snap or get short with your partner's annoying quirks. And remember, just because something he or she does bothers you does not mean you have the right to ask your partner to stop doing it. If the behavior is relatively normal, harmless, and you are the only one annoyed, it is unfair to blame the problem on your partner and act like his or her behavior is inferior to yours. Think of it as strengthening your tolerance muscle, and watch it reap dividends.

I have said it before, but it is worth repeating: be careful with your tone. Tone of voice can send all sorts of unintended or triggering messages. Tone of voice can be the verbal equivalent of an eye roll or a "whatever"; it can also effectively express love and concern. Be mindful to whom you are speaking and how much you value that person. Be patient about a partner's decision-making process, even though it may be different or slower than yours. Be patient with the pace at which your partner learns something that is important to you. Remember that all of us are still learning and that we bring different strengths and weaknesses.

POINTS TO REMEMBER

- When we marry, we effectively promise more than what we state in our vows. We promise to respect our spouse in ways large and small, through being thoughtful about how what we do affects them.

- It is easy to fall into bad marital habits as time passes and you become used to each other. Do not let this overshadow the positive aspects of your partner and relationship.

- Bad habits can include failing to listen, being too critical, or reflexively rejecting any complaint offered by your partner. Be mindful of your bad habits, and remain open to your partner's request for change.

- The failure to remember why we fell in love initially can lead us to take our partner for granted, to fail to praise them, to show affection, or to take their side when they need us to. Remain active in your efforts to cherish your partner.

For more resources, go to:
www.DrAnneMalec.com

CHAPTER FIVE:

Being a Good Roommate

Relationships require a variety of skills to stay connected and on track with our partners. One aspect of a healthy relationship is being a good roommate. Just like with your college roommate, living together will be easier and more pleasant if you coordinate everyday tasks and living preferences with your spouse. Coordination requires treating each other fairly as partners and being open and respectful about your needs.

It is easy for bad habits to creep into a relationship over time. A year or two into a relationship, partners can feel like it is "safe" enough to ease up on their best behavior, hoping the love is strong enough for a partner to overlook bad habits. The gradual easing up is triggered by the belief that it is now safe to show our "true selves" without running the risk of our partners abandoning us. Remember back when you were dating and you would not have dreamed of allowing your sweetheart to see how messy you were or how infrequently you did laundry. When you begin to feel a deeper attachment to a romantic partner, surface-level worries recede, and you may even take pride in how well your partner accepts these character traits. However, it is important to remain considerate of your partner sharing a living space with you, and open communication can reduce the likelihood of either partner building resentment about bad habits gone awry.

A common complaint from couples living together is dissatisfaction with the division of labor. When I ask couples how they decided on the current division of labor, I often receive blank stares. Rarely was such a conversation had, with partners instead making a nonverbal pact for their living arrangement. How do household tasks or patterns get "assigned" without verbally communicating about them? Some duties are established based upon likes or dislikes, how your parents divided housework tasks, how much your parents did for you while you were growing up, and dating behaviors that become permanent expectations.

Perhaps early on in your relationship you wanted to exhibit the nurturing parts of your personality, so you frequently cooked for your new boyfriend or girlfriend. Or maybe you wanted to show a romantic interest your financial success by picking up the bill at every shared meal. It is not unusual during this period to exhibit traits consistent with the norms for your gender. Should the relationship become permanent, you may expect your partner to continue these behaviors and feel compelled to keep up the tasks you initially assigned to yourself. Maintaining these behaviors may stem from a desire to avoid feeling like you have enticed your partner through a "bait and switch" in which you attracted your partner by exhibiting certain characteristics and behaviors, but then once the relationship feels like a sure thing, you stop engaging in those appealing behaviors. However, disgruntlement can develop if either of you feels that certain tasks are expected of you just because you did them in the early days. Talk to your partner about what each of you perceives to be fair in the sharing of responsibilities. Tasks grow and change over the years, so be willing to continue the conversation.

Through my clinical and personal experience, I compiled a list of hints for being a good roommate when you share a living space:

- Clean up after yourself.

- Put your dishes in the dishwasher.

- If you have a closet, hang your coat in it.

- Do not use all the hot water.

- Keep your bodily functions private (not everyone thinks it is funny or interesting).

- Always text or call if you are running late. If you habitually run late and keep your partner waiting, work to change your behavior. It feels disrespectful to the more punctual partner.

- Take your turn communicating with the child-care professionals and teachers.

- If you eat together at home, you should share the meal preparation. When the other party cooks, you should do the dishes and take out the trash if it needs doing.

- Just because your mother did the laundry does not mean you should assume your wife will, too—or that just because your father took care of the yard means it is your husband's job. Discuss who does each task and reach an equitable division.

- Going to bed at the same time creates opportunities for cuddling.

- Set your alarm clock, and do not rely on your spouse to wake you up. Be considerate of how often you push "snooze" if you get up before your partner in the morning.

- Call and schedule your own appointments: medical, dental, hair, and so on.

- The car's driver selects the route and chooses the music.

- If your driving style makes your spouse anxious (something I hear a lot of women say), do not dismiss your spouse's fears. Make adjustments to your speed while driving together (imagine how you would feel if *your* request was ignored).

- Never tell your spouse you think he or she is crazy and do not diagnose them with a personality disorder (especially if you are a therapist).

- If you ask for your partner's help in doing something and it is important that it be completed by a certain time or date, tell him or her when and why when asking for help. This way he or she can commit to it (or not). Do not ask your partner for help without making the timing clear and then resent him or her for not helping when you need it.

- Do not expect your partner to keep track of all the important dates for your family, to buy all the birthday and holiday gifts, or to send the cards.

- Show an active interest in what your partner likes (it warms my heart to hear my husband ask what time *Iron Chef* is on).

- Take turns changing the cat litter, even if you only inherited the cat through marriage.

- Offer to help with snow shoveling and yard maintenance, even if you think it is his job.

- Be considerate of the difference between personal and shared space.

- Give your partner space to decompress once he or she arrives home. Some people can make the transition from home to work during the commute, but others may need time and space after arriving home. If this sounds like your partner, give him or her space to read the paper, check scores, play a video game, review the iPad, check emails, and so on. It usually does not take long, and it is worth the time to have a relaxed spouse who is physically *and* emotionally present.

- Remember, part of what makes for good roommates is regularly getting out of the "room." Make sure that you plan to spend couple time together away from home. Plan regular date nights, and place them on your schedule. Do not place the full responsibility for planning these, making the reservation, and calling a sitter on just one of you. If you share the fun, then share the planning.

How many of these considerations do you already show your partner? Work with your partner to add or subtract from this list and make more applicable "good roommate" guidelines for your relationship. It can be a helpful reference when you are feeling frustrated, and it holds both of you accountable to your agreement to be a good roommate.

ROOMMATE SUGGESTIONS WHEN A
PARTNER TRAVELS FREQUENTLY

If you have a partner who frequently travels for his or her job, you face additional challenges for maintaining healthy boundaries. Traveling for business is stressful for both members in a relationship. The traveler feels stressed from being away from the family's love and support and the familiarity of home, and the spouse left behind is stressed by not having someone to share in the work. But with the modern technology available, staying connected has never been easier. Here are some suggestions for staying connected when one of you travels for business:

- **Recognize that the stay-at-home partner has a "routine" when at home without the traveling partner.** This routine includes how he or she parents while alone, such as morning, dinner, and bedtime routines for the kids. If you are the traveling partner, upon your return, be mindful of the routine and try not to disrupt it too much, as it could create frustration with your partner. The best way to learn about the existence of a routine is to ask your partner about it and then figure out how to smooth the transition.

- **Make sure your partner knows your location.** This sounds obvious, but due to the pace of modern life, partners of frequently traveling spouses do not always know where the traveler is. Anxiety lessens with certainty. Create a shared calendar, and keep your travel plans up to date. Use the same calendar to keep track of important dates, such as birthdays, school events, and family time. Make a sincere effort to respect family time by scheduling work travel around important dates.

- **Make use of video conferencing.** In a previous chapter, I discussed the need to create time to check in daily and connect with one another—preferably face to face. Looking at each other, eye to eye, creates a closer connection. Whether you prefer Skype, FaceTime, or another application, take advantage of available technology to stay in contact.

- **Relationships need smooth takeoffs and landings.** Routines lessen anxiety. Make an effort to start and end your day together via phone or Skype, etc. A quick phone call to say "Good night, I love you" to your partner builds a secure and loving connection, as well as a better night's sleep.

- **Maintain shared interests despite the distance.** Read the same book or keep up with one another's favorite television show. Discuss current events in your daily check-in and share the little things that bind you together, such as what your boss said about your client proposal, what gossip you picked up on Facebook or from talking to your neighbor, the funny thing your child said, and so on.

- **Occasionally arrange to travel with your partner.** Turn business trips into short getaways, and use earned miles or points to visit new places together.

- **Ensure that the partner at home has adequate support in your absence.** It is not uncommon for the stay-at-home partner to feel abandoned and overwhelmed by the responsibility of maintaining the home, children, and pets while working a full-time job. Utilize your support network: call on family members and friends to help out your spouse or consider hiring a cleaning service, dinner delivery service, or dog walker to lighten the burden. For the partner that travels, make sure you express your appreciation for all that the other does to keep the home fires burning.

- **Appreciation goes both ways.** Partners who frequently travel for work rarely find it glamorous, exciting, or restful. Business travel can be a series of hours spent waiting in airports, sleeping in uncomfortable beds, day-long meetings, and "road food." Remember that you are a team, and express appreciation for the traveler's hard work and sacrifice. It might feel to the stay-at-home partner that the traveling spouse has the better deal, but this is not necessarily true and can be a dangerous assumption. Your partner would probably rather be home with you.

- **Transition home smoothly.** The first 30 minutes upon arriving home from work is prime conflict time for overstressed couples. The first thing on the agenda for the at-home partner may be, "Thank God you're home so you can give me some help." The first thing on the traveler's mind is often, "Thank God I'm home so I can finally relax." Give each other some decompression time, and be sure to carve out time for couple reconnection after the kids are in bed.

- **Topics for your check-in calls.** Frequent traveling manifests the illusion that there is no good time to talk or discuss what is going on within the family, and the at-home partner may struggle about whether to raise a complicated issue, such as feeling overwhelmed or unappreciated. Despite modern technology, remote discussions are probably not the ideal time to discuss issues that could lead to disagreement or conflict or that will require an extended discussion to solve them. If such discussions are necessary, save them for when you are both at home and work together to find a time where you can both give the topic its due consideration. If possible, make your daily check-in time free of conflict and triggering topics.

• **Remind your partner that you are thinking of him or her.** Utilize text messages and emails for short and sweet communication, and save deeper topics for face-to-face or voice-to-voice time. Such seemingly small efforts in communicating that your partner is in your thoughts can go a long way in preserving an intimate connection.

Understand and accept that marital love is not unconditional—that there are conditions each of us will find unacceptable in life overall and that they apply both to your relationship and your physical surroundings. Follow the Golden Rule: treat your spouse as you want to be treated. It applies equally to your living space. Treat your home space the way you would like your partner to treat it. And if specific habits are bothersome, discuss them respectfully with your mate.

POINTS TO REMEMBER

- Sharing space with other people, whether roommates or partners, requires being mindful of their needs and preferences.

- You may be irritated by some habits your partner has. Remember that you, too, are not free of irritating habits. Choose your battles wisely, being cognizant that you cannot win them all, nor should you try.

- Finding a spouse does not mean you acquired a live-in cook, housekeeper, or gardener. Discuss what needs to be done to keep the household running, and establish a plan for splitting the work that is fair to both of you.

- If you travel, make time to connect and check in with your spouse on a regular basis. Work to keep check-ins free of conflict.

For more resources, go to:
www.DrAnneMalec.com

CHAPTER SIX:

Money Matters

Given my background in accounting and business, it may not be surprising that the money chapter is the longest one in this book. In addition to providing traditional couples and individual counseling, I also provide financial therapy. I frequently see money problems create discord and unhappiness in relationships. In all marriages, whether both partners work, one spouse stays home to care for children, or in blended families, money often takes center stage in couple conflict. Like most other areas of conflict, frequent communication and formulating a plan for how to address the financial situation allows many, if not most, issues to be adequately and respectfully resolved.

All of us bring into romantic relationships a belief structure about how our joint financial life will play out, and rarely do these beliefs perfectly match with our partner's beliefs. Our beliefs are created, often subconsciously, with influence from our families, society, gender-related expectations, and friends. Each partner will bring a different set of beliefs and expectations, but rarely do partners fully communicate these expectations. Often, neither partner knows what the other expects or how his or her partner's beliefs and expectations will manifest in the relationship. The tendency to let financial management unfold without prior planning and mutual agreement leads money to be a top contender in couple conflict. Reiterating a central theme in the book: communication is a must.

Every couple faces a unique financial situation. No book can address every potential issue you may come across during your life together, especially in only one chapter! What does apply to every couple is the need to create an emotionally safe and respectful communication space to effectively understand each other's perspectives and reach a resolution.

COMMON FINANCIAL STRUGGLES AND PROPOSED SOLUTIONS

Every couple has to determine how their joint and individual expenses will be shared. Family expenses usually include: rent or mortgage, property taxes, car payments, gas and repair, utilities, cable, cell phones, house cleaning expenses, children's tuition, children's extracurricular activities, spouse's tuition, clothing, couple entertainment, travel/vacations, co-pays for health care, exercise or health club expenses, home repair, health and auto insurance, pet care, babysitting/nanny/child care, groceries, etc. However, most partners also have individual interests or hobbies that require financial support. Among many couples there can be disagreement about the personal spending choices of the other, often causing frequent conflict. One way to avoid this is to add to your family budget a line item for your personal monthly budget.

Each partner's personal monthly budget is an agreed-upon amount that is spent freely and about which your partner should not question or impose judgment. *Your partner has no voice in how you spend it* (assuming it is legal and consistent with your marriage vows). These funds cover personal items such as coffee, lunches, bar tabs, pedicures, poker night, purses, and salon costs. The personal monthly budget reduces the chances of having stressful discussions such as "You bought more shoes? Do you really need more shoes?" or "You've joined another fantasy football league?" or "Why did you pick up the tab with your coworkers?" If you do not want to spend the funds in your personal account, great, then save it. Having an agreed personal monthly budget helps minimize financial tension between the couple and gives each partner a sense of financial autonomy within the boundaries of the family's finances.

Some spouses combine their money and keep it in one account while others keep separate credit cards, checking, savings, and investment accounts. Regardless of your financial structure, sooner or later partners must discuss spending habits or priorities and who pays what bills. A common practice in dividing expenses for couples is based on your proportion of the joint income. For example, if you earn 55 percent of the family income, you pay 55 percent of the family expenses.

However, a simple approach like this may not work if the dynamics are more complex due to an unequal division of household tasks or pre-relationship obligations. It is neither inappropriate nor unusual for a couple to have a discussion about what gets deducted from one's individual income before sharing the family expenses. Some couples may want to consider contributions made in-kind when dividing expenses. For example, hypothetical couple George and Gretchen earn a combined $100,000 per year. If each partner earns $50,000 but Gretchen spends twice the amount of time on cooking and cleaning than George, there should be a recognition of this time when family expenses get divided. The partner contributing more to housework should have a smaller share of the family expenses.

Pre-relationship obligations also complicate a shared marital budget. These expenses include:

- Student loan debt

- Medical bills

- Child support

- College tuition accounts

- Credit card debt from before your marriage

- Alimony/maintenance for a former spouse

- Providing financial assistance for parents or other adult family member.

If you have these added expenses in your relationship, consider sharing current family expenses based on your disposable income after deducting any pre-relationship obligations.

Every couple should have regular budget meetings, which can be added as a part of your weekly check-in meetings, to allow for a full discussion of all money matters. If you have trouble having these on an impromptu basis, schedule them monthly (or weekly, if warranted). Some topics requiring routine discussions include:

- Changes in family income

- Family budget changes

- Upcoming household related expenses

- Wants/needs for each of you related to the spending for your home, autos, or other significant expenses

- Vacation plans and associated expenses

- Tax-related issues

- Changes to your personal monthly budget

- Kids' upcoming expenses
- Retirement savings

If you feel uneducated about money, read about it. Through learning, your anxiety will decrease, your confidence increase, and your marital conflict lessen (see www.drannemalec.com for a list of resources). For additional help, consider consulting with a professional financial advisor.

It is important for partners to agree on their definition of family income. For example, should it include child support payments, received inheritance, premarital assets, investment income, or bonuses? There are as many different answers as there are couples. The important thing is to be open and honest in discussing these issues—ideally before the marriage—and come to an agreement. If you need help, contact a financial or marriage and family therapist.

Another area of potential conflict is when one partner makes a financial commitment that affects both parties. In situations where both parties and any children can be affected, neither one of you should make a significant long-term financial commitment unless you are both in agreement. It is important that you discuss and reach agreement on what constitutes "significant." This, too, varies by couple and situation. To a family surviving on a very limited income, almost any unnecessary expenditure can be financially devastating. For high-income partners, new golf clubs may cause no added stress on the family's financial situation. By talking through what is and is not financially significant, partners can avoid ugly surprises and make sure they are on the same page about spending and saving priorities.

Couples may want to set a standard that if a partner is considering a purchase that is over a set amount, he or she will consult with the other before spending. For instance, if you agreed on a spending limit of $200, you will consult with your partner before making a purchase over that amount. This guideline pertains to expenses considered to be family expenses and does not apply to your personal monthly budget.

COMMON CAUSES OF MARITAL FINANCIAL CONFLICT:

Spouses Who Fail to Take Responsibility for Family Finances.

When one partner has to carry most of the financial burden, it can thrust that partner into an almost *parental* role over the other. The partner choosing to remain uninformed about money matters is sending a message that he or she cannot cope with being involved in financial decision-making or in being financially accountable. For some individuals, any talk of money creates anxiety. But deliberately choosing not to have a voice in the budgeting, spending, saving, or investing of your family's income is a precarious position to take. You are essentially giving away control over your financial life and risk becoming the "child" to the "parent" partner. An unintended danger in this dynamic is that the couple may begin relating similarly in other aspects of the relationship, whereby one partner holds more power/control than the other, which can create resentment.

I am very much a believer in the importance of both partners being fully informed and responsible for their individual and family finances. Partners who rationalize their lack of involvement in money matters commonly say, "Well, he (or she) is better at it and likes doing it." While this may be true, it is still irresponsible to be uninvolved in this vital aspect of your life and marriage, and it may put undue pressure on the other partner. When one partner solely manages the family finances, he or she often feels burdened, like the "bad guy" who has to say no to requests for spending or has to make the tough choices. This can lead to money trouble if the financially accountable spouse does not like saying no to spending requests because it causes him or her to feel like an inadequate provider.

Spouses Who Control or Micromanage the Spending of Their Partners. If you earn more than your partner, have a stay-at-home spouse, or believe you are simply better equipped to manage the family finances, be careful about claiming the right to be the family's financial decision maker. Within a partnership, neither partner controls the veto pen. Controlling the spending of your partner may lead to a situation where your spouse feels like his or her needs are unimportant, which can breed feelings of resentment, insecurity, and depression. You are an equal partner to your spouse, not a parent to them. If a couple decides that one partner will stay at home to care for the children, work toward an academic degree, or pursue another goal, it is because both partners jointly made this decision. The decision and the work done outside of a traditional workplace should be valued for what it is, a contribution to the family.

You never want to create a dynamic where your partner feels like a second-class citizen in your relationship. Micromanaging a spouse's spending or passing judgment on him or her for what you deem to be materialistic purchases could create a situation where your spouse hides spending. It is safe to assume your partner will resent your efforts to control his or her behavior. Just because your spouse likes beautiful things, big-screen televisions, or nice cars does not mean related purchases are materialistic, wasteful, or indicate the existence of questionable values. Both parties should keep in mind that some purchases are made not just for shelter and safety but because they make the other party happy. You may want to consider creating a personal monthly budget to limit the controlling tendencies of the micro-managing partner.

An important caveat: should you believe your partner's spending is a reaction to an underlying emotional issue like depression, anxiety, emptiness, or poor self-esteem, make your concerns known in a loving way. If you fear that your partner is hiding debt or spending, you must also make these concerns known. These overspending risks can be minimized with the use of a personal monthly budget and financial openness in your individual and joint lives.

Resentment about Pre-Relationship Obligations.

It is important for both parties to realize that there may be strong emotions associated with pre-relationship financial obligations. Paying a former spouse alimony or child support is the reality for millions of couples in which one or both partners is divorced. It is also increasingly common for young couples to bring education debt into a new marriage. It is helpful to view these obligations as a legal requirement and not optional. In the vast majority of cases, you will have known about the financial obligation for as long as you have known your partner. Try not to let your frustration become a cause of conflict or tension between the two of you. Talk through your financial concerns in an open and nonjudgmental manner, striving to understand your partner's goals in meeting these obligations. Remain aware that you may need to bite your tongue more often than not in regards to these expenditures. In some ways, complaining about a pre-existing legal obligation that you knew about is like complaining about your partner's height or eye color. The obligation is simply a part of the package for which you signed on.

Support for a former spouse can be an especially sensitive topic. The sensitivity and discomfort often stem from feeling that an ex-partner is benefiting from income that you feel should be devoted to you and your partner's new family. No doubt about it, this is difficult to accept, especially if there is ongoing acrimony from the previous relationship. Money spent on child support can also create strain in a relationship if it diminishes the resources available for children born into the new marriage. Due to guilt created during the divorce, some parents may be especially sensitive to discussions about money spent on child support. Providing money for children from a prior marriage can absolve a partner of some of his or her regret and remorse about how the divorce proceeded. This is especially true for the party who initiated the divorce. Share openly with your partner the emotional benefit you feel in being able to provide for your first family.

As previously stated, a partner is almost always aware of, or should have been aware of, a spouse's financial obligation to his or her children and ex-spouse prior to committing to the new relationship. Discussing these issues early in your engagement and determining a workable plan will serve your relationship well.

Here are a few tips on how to avoid a recurring monthly conflict about pre-relationship obligations:

- Arrange for the financial transaction to be handled only by the spouse with the commitment.

- Transfer the payment directly from a payroll account.

- Maintain a separate bank account for child support expenses.

- Inform your partner of any changes to your financial obligations.

- *Do not hide* any unexpected expenses related to your children from your prior relationship.

Stay-at-Home Moms.

Most modern couples are dual-income earners. According to the Bureau of Labor Statistics, 62.4 percent of married couples with children aged 6–17 and 54.6 percent of married couples with children under six years old consist of partners who both engage in paid work.[13] However, there are still many couples that make the decision for one partner to stay home, usually to take care of children. While this decision may make a lot of sense initially, it should be revisited at least once a year to address any feelings that change or new financial concerns.

One reason to frequently revisit this decision is because research indicates that the longer a woman is out of the workforce, the longer it can take to find a job. Sylvia Ann Hewitt of the Center for Work-Life Policy reports, "two-thirds of all women who quit their career to raise children are seeking to reenter professional life and finding it exceedingly difficult."[14] Transitioning back into the paid labor force may be more challenging than previously thought, a reality that can put additional financial and career stress on a marriage. While 74 percent of stay-at-home moms successfully reenter the workforce, only 40 percent of those return to full-time professional jobs, 24 percent take part-time jobs, and about 9 percent become self-employed.[15]

Women leaving the workforce to care for children may have every intention of returning to paid work, but the economic hit to their earning power can happen quickly and be long-lasting. This "mommy tax" can add up to a lifetime penalty of more than $1 million for a college-educated American woman who has children and leaves the workforce to be a stay-at-home mom.[16] The "mommy tax" is manifested in reduced earnings, pensions, social security benefits, 401(k) contributions, and health-care benefits. The reduced lifetime earnings for stay-at-home mothers should be a consideration when determining the best child-care options for your family. Even more concerning, when a marriage ends, a woman's standard of living drops by 36 percent, whereas a man's standard of living rises by 28 percent.[17] This divorce effect on women likely results from a combination of factors: being a stay-at-home parent, the "mommy tax," earning less than your former spouse, and mothers traditionally getting custody of their children (thereby having fewer hours available for work).

Other data for consideration in determining the best child-care arrangement for your family: women are almost twice as likely as men to live below the poverty line during retirement, with a median income of approximately $16,000 a year—about $11,000 less than men of the same age. Women earn and save less over their lifetimes, but they tend to live longer. On average, women work 12 years less than men do over the course of their careers, mostly due to raising kids or caring for an ill spouse or aging parents.[18]

There is more at stake for stay-at-home parents than reduced income: diminished self-confidence, a potential loss of purpose or direction, and being seen differently through the eyes of one's partner are common side effects. When you met your spouse, you were probably financially independent. Your career focus and ambition may have been one of the things your partner found attractive about you. When you choose to stay at home to care for children, you make a trade-off. Becoming financially dependent on your partner changes your relationship, and it may even change how you feel about yourself. You may not feel challenged, appreciated, respected, or intellectually stimulated. Some of the topics you and your spouse had previously connected on may fall away, as much of your time is spent with your children and much of his time at the office. It is not unusual for partners to feel as though they grow apart during these years if one spouse is working and the other is at home.

I was first introduced to this data about the financial losses of stay-at-home mothers while completing a master's thesis. The information astounded me. I want to share it with you not to scare or anger but to inform so that you can make the best decisions as an individual, a parent, and a spouse. Some couples may determine that it is best for their family that someone stay at home to care for a child or children, and I do not intend to criticize this lifestyle choice. Women reading this book may disagree with these comments, but my point in sharing them with you is not to show any disrespect for your family structure or propose a family reorganization for contented stay-at-home mothers. My hope is to make couples more aware of the risks involved before deciding that a woman will stay at home to care for the children. It is important to remain mindful of any potential short-term and long-term financial drawbacks and the impact this family structure can have on a marriage. Each couple needs to determine a family structure that works best for both partners today, tomorrow, and well into the future.

Stay-at-Home Dads.

There appears to be tremendous resistance to societal acceptance of stay-at-home fathers, with most men feeling pressured to define themselves by their ability to be a provider for their wives and families. Gender norms influence one's definition of what it means to be a man or a woman, and they can directly or indirectly affect partners' perceptions of what is expected or accepted in a relationship or family. Even though the expectation of the man/father/husband being the main provider is an entrenched aspect of American life, the data point to big changes ahead. It is estimated that the number of couples with stay-at-home fathers increased from 3.4 percent in 1999 to 5.6 percent in 2009,[19] with as many as 2.2 million stay-at-home dads in 2010.[20] While this is a growing trend, culturally we are slower to catch up. Pew Social Trends found that 51 percent of respondents indicated a belief that children are better off if a mother is home and does not hold a job, while only 8 percent said the same about the impact of stay-at-home fathers.[21] The lack of respect and support facing stay-at-home dads adds obstacles to maintaining this arrangement in a marriage.

If this is the setup in your family, your husband is a pioneer in this emerging trend, and he may feel inadequate for not living up to the cultural expectation of being a "provider." Even if a man is comfortable with his decision to stay home to care for the children, he may still feel negatively judged by his family, friends, or former colleagues. Perceived judgment or lack of support can add unique stressors to the marital relationship. Chesley (2011) found that breadwinning moms spoke of the guilt and jealousy that they felt when comparing their parenting time to that of their stay-at-home husbands, and moms felt constrained in their choices because of the family's dependence on their income. Because society perpetuates the stereotype of men being the traditional financial providers, stay-at-home dads report feeling conflicted about the decision due to pressure from their masculine ideals, their wives' expectations, and societal messages. While a woman may very much enjoy the earning power and sense of being financially independent, being the sole breadwinner is probably not something that she bargained for going into her marriage. Similarly, men may rarely imagine a life where they are financially dependent on or outearned by their wives.

It helps to talk directly about what one expects from the other so as to avoid harmful assumptions or biases that prevent families from developing a structure that works for both partners (rather than a structure that *society* deems appropriate). For many couples, this is new and unexpected territory that requires openness to discussion and a willingness to adapt. Budget discussions and financial problem-solving are particularly important for the working wife and stay-at-home-husband couple because there is often a lot of emotional and psychological baggage that comes with a male relinquishing his provider status to become the at-home parent. Couples need to be careful not to create a sense of shame around the man's financial dependence. Making it okay and emotionally safe for a man to talk about feelings of shame, fear, or anxiety, and for a breadwinning wife to share her concerns about emasculating or dominating her partner, allows the couple to forge ahead in creating a system that works for *their* family, no matter the outside noise.

The smart thing to do is to talk about and fully explore your options for managing your finances before having children, and figure out a system that works for you. Allow you and your partner the flexibility to adjust the structure if the current setup fosters significant stress or resentment after a trial period. Remember that you are in this together and that this is new ground for both of you. If you need help with the conversation, contact an MFT or FT. You may also benefit from reviewing the book *When She Makes More* by Farnoosh Torabi.

Wives Outearning Husbands.

With increasing frequency in my practice and our culture at large, I see couples where women outearn their husbands. Data from 2012 indicate that 38.1 percent of wives earn more than their husbands as compared with 10.8 percent in 1960 and 24 percent in 1980.[23] For many couples, this setup functions well, with males reacting positively to this modern development. But for others, it can create anxiety and discomfort for both the wives and their husbands.

Many modern couples are trying to find their way through this complex issue, and it is not easy. For some women earning more than their husbands, research has found that they give greater deference to their husbands to not appear dominating. And even though power is frequently associated with income, women do not report an increase in power within the home due to their superior earning power.[24] Supporting these findings is research from the University of Chicago that reveals that women and men continue making decisions to maintain feminine and masculine identity expectations and norms in the face of a nontraditional earning structure.[25] In practice, this can mean a woman takes on more housework and child care and potentially passes on employment opportunities where she could outearn her husband. Couples with this survival strategy were found to be less satisfied with their marriages and had higher rates of divorce.

If you were raised in a home where the male was the main breadwinner, you would understandably see a traditional arrangement as "normal" and probably believe that the same would be true in your marriage. If you are a man facing the reality of your female partner being the lead breadwinner, this can strike at the core of your masculine identity because of our culture's tendency to equate manhood with earning capacity. Farnoosh Torabi, writing in *When She Makes More*, reports that when a wife outearns her husband, in an effort to maintain gender norms and reduce anxiety, women tend to take on more housework and child care than their husbands. Concurrently, husbands holding traditional gender values may be unaware of the imbalance if it is not directly communicated. This can lead to unintended and self-induced resentment in women who feel burdened and unappreciated for their hard work. Tarobi also reports that in marriages where wives outearn their husbands, both partners are susceptible to the following psychological and sexual side effects: impotency, lack of intimacy, and reduced attraction.[26]

I interpret these findings to mean that the often-misguided efforts to maintain gender norms within these relationships eventually become too difficult and the marriages founder. If a higher-earning woman tries to maintain traditional gender norms within her marriage so that she feels more comfortable and like a "traditional woman," she is most likely taking on more than she can manage. Trying to blend the demands of modern life with the expectations of a traditional marriage is the road to burnout. This situation may be created because she feels uncomfortable asking her partner for more help due to a fear of emasculating him, or perhaps she feels guilty about earning more and is trying to protect his ego from being asked to do what has been traditionally known as "women's work." The data suggest that greater income does not lead to a less stressful home life for women. The way to tackle this problem is to ask your partner for what you need. Talk about your concerns of taking on too much in order to avoid feeling like you are too dominating or emasculating. Tell your partner when and where you need more help, and problem-solve together. Fight the impulse to meet the expectations of outdated gender norms.

For marriages that end in divorce due to a failure to balance a nontraditional earning structure with traditional gender norms, I hypothesize that equity theory (from chapter 3) is at play. When one partner is the main breadwinner and does the heavier share of child care and housework, the situation will not wear well on the relationship. In order for this family structure to succeed, something has got to give; there needs to be a fairer division of household labor and child care. If there is an unaddressed imbalance in the individual contribution of each partner, this inevitably leads to resentment. Just as it is unfair to expect a husband to earn the majority of the family income and do the majority of household tasks and child care, it is equally unfair to expect this of a wife. The way to successfully make it through this modern day scenario is to communicate, balance, and rebalance as often as is necessary.

Without family role models providing healthy examples of how to navigate this reality, you are left to figure it out on your own. You are driving without a working GPS, but you are not alone in the car. Like every other emotionally complex topic that couples face, this issue can become less disruptive the more feelings and thoughts are shared. Neither one of you may have predicted the difficulty associated with a wife earning more, but if it bothers either one of you, you cannot deny your feelings and expect there to be no consequences. Address the elephant in the room before it takes up all the space. Start by talking about it. It is okay to say, "It feels weird that I am earning more money than you. How does it feel to you?" You may even benefit from talking about the research findings and sharing your thoughts about them. Create the time and space for ongoing dialogue. Develop your own family norms, modeling for your children how to be successful in a modern marriage.

Responding to Your Partner's Financial SOS.

Due to changes in the job market and the economy, it is not uncommon for partners to find it necessary to increase their family's income. Requests for increased family income cannot be addressed quickly and painlessly. Returning to the workforce after years spent at home is fraught with challenges; a spouse may not have kept skills and professional contacts, and he or she may not know what type of work is available at this stage in life.

No matter how much sense it made at the time, these spouses can feel boxed in by a decision jointly made years earlier to stay home. Reentry after years out of the job market can feel daunting, intimidating, and scary. It might feel very unexpected and unsettling for your partner to bring up this drastic change, and that is normal. But when your partner makes this request, you have a responsibility and an obligation to listen and understand what motivated the request. Is it a financial concern? Does your spouse fear that he or she may be at risk of losing a job? Are there inadequate savings for college and retirement? This request may feel like it came out of left field, but there is likely a good reason for your partner to broach such a serious issue. It might require a lot of soul-searching and thoughtful discussion in exploring possible opportunities.

If you are the breadwinning partner who wants to see your spouse back in the workforce, understand how intimidating that prospect might feel, and find a way to help. Like the rest of your relationship, this requires a team effort. A spouse returning to the workforce after years at home will need the unwavering support of a partner, as he or she is likely dealing with anxiety, self-doubt, and insecurity. Know that your partner will need your empathy and support throughout the process, along with your assistance in updating a resume, networking, or brainstorming different opportunities. Do what you can to make the return to the workforce as smooth as possible, which will probably include your needing to take on more child care and household responsibilities.

Financial Infidelity.

Financial infidelity occurs when a spouse leads a secret financial life. Researchers from the National Endowment for Financial Education report that close to one third of those who have combined their finances with a partner admit to hiding cash, purchases, a bank account, or a credit card. Further, 13 percent of survey participants report having lied to their partners about their income or debt.[27] Financial infidelity can also stem from gambling debts, a shopping or collecting addiction, or even a drug or pornography addiction. It may also be related to a naïve unwillingness to face the reality of placing limits on family spending.

Often partners become ensnared in financial infidelity because they are afraid to have honest conversations with their spouses about the realities of their financial situation or destructive habits. The financially unfaithful partner rationalizes not being honest with his or her partner because of a fear that if he or she reveals the truth, the unsuspecting spouse will be angry, which will only make the situation worse. If you cannot or will not discuss these types of issues with your partner, I suggest you discuss them with a therapist before you dig a hole too deep for your marriage to survive. Some people justify secret financial dealings to themselves by saying that they are "protecting" the spouse from worry. But hiding debts, bills, or spending habits from a partner to protect him or her is more about protecting yourself from your partner's reaction.

True partnership requires complete honesty about spending and debt. If you find yourself withholding information from your partner, it may be that you are trying to protect yourself from feeling as though you have somehow failed your partner as a provider. You are living beyond your means instead of saying, "We cannot afford this." Talk to each other often. Accept your responsibilities for financial openness and honesty.

PRENUPTIAL AGREEMENTS

Prenuptial agreements are an increasingly common aspect of modern marriages. A 2013 survey of the American Academy of Matrimonial Lawyers[28] reported 63 percent of divorce attorneys seeing an increase in prenuptial agreements (prenups) in the past three years. Forty-six percent noted an increase in the number of women requesting prenups. The increased popularity of prenups may be due to an increase in the age of people in first marriages—when they have assets, student loan or credit card debt, or business partnerships—and to more people remarrying after failure of a prior marriage.

No one entering a marriage wants to believe that there is a significant risk it will fail or that your partner is focused on preparing for this potentiality. Yet statistics tell us there is a significant chance that a first marriage will fail. If this is a second, third, or fourth marriage, there is an even greater chance it will not last.[29] Having a prenuptial agreement about how you are going to treat each other in the event of a divorce makes a lot of sense in the face of these statistics.

Broaching the Topic.

For many reasons, the topic of a prenuptial agreement can make romantic partners very uncomfortable. A prospective spouse proposing a prenup might give rise to anxiety that he or she believes the marriage might not last. It may also make you feel as if, should your marriage not last, you are not trusted enough to work out a fair dissolution. You might ask yourself: "Why is he saying this? Is he unsure? What is he afraid of?"

I can certainly understand the unromantic quality of a prenup and can empathize with both sides of the issue. My husband had assets and children at the time of our marriage, but he did not request that I sign one. I am confident that it would have upset me had he asked, as it probably would have made me question whether he doubted our relationship and, more significantly, if he trusted me. In retrospect, having now built a business of my own, the person I am today would have understood the request. From his perspective, he would have known that marriages are not foolproof and that in making decisions about the division of assets, judges sometimes rule against your best interests.

If a prenup is desired by one or both partners, when is the best time to raise the issue? Ideally, after the engagement but prior to the day before the wedding. It makes sense to work out an agreement when you both feel the most loving toward each other and not angry or resentful. Try not to be fearful in bringing it up—just have good reasons for wanting a prenup, and clearly explain those reasons.

If your partner proposes a prenuptial agreement, it may help to think of it as an insurance policy. Customarily we take out insurance to protect us in the event of something catastrophic happening; we do not want such an event to bankrupt us. The most common provisions in prenups deal with economic issues: treatment of property owned individually, alimony/spousal maintenance, and division of marital property.[30]

While a prenup can sound unromantic, and it may be painful to think that your partner does not trust in you, considering the statistics on divorce, a prenup serves as a safety net for you and your future family.

If your partner resists signing a prenup, it does not necessarily signify anything negative about your relationship, it may mean that he or she finds your request too pessimistic or business-like. Your partner may be unwilling or unable to determine before the marriage what he or she will agree to if the relationship fails. Dedicate the time for each of you to communicate your fears and concerns. There is no right or wrong on this topic. You will each have a unique perspective that needs to be heard.

It is not unusual for couples to bring professional assistance into this discussion. A marriage and family therapist can provide structure and a safe space to talk about it. Even if you both agree on having a prenup, an MFT can assist with the discussion of what each party wants the agreement to cover and why. The therapist's office provides emotional safety and a supportive environment in which to share your thoughts, feelings, fears, and anxieties. A therapist can provide a much-needed perspective, normalizing each of your points of view.

While I have high regard for the legal profession, attorneys typically represent one party or the other. This makes for a vastly different conversation—with one party seeming to be on offense and the other on defense. Consider working out the content in a therapist's office and then hiring attorneys to draft the contract to which you both agree.

How to Talk about It.

Discussion about potential divorce will feel unromantic. So will the pragmatic aspect of how you will divide your assets and liabilities and arrange to pay alimony or maintenance. Therefore, it is very important to have this discussion in a way that you can actively show your partner how much you love him or her. Come to the discussion from a very loving and supportive place: how will you treat this person whom you love deeply should your relationship founder?

One proactive way to begin this discussion is with a parallel discussion of the compact the two of you will make to ensure your marriage thrives. The prenup becomes a contingency plan for a worst-case scenario. The plan to make the marriage work should include what you will each do to prioritize your relationship as a couple, allow for and continue to seek personal development and fulfillment, manage and communicate about family finances, and develop a couple strategy for solving difficult problems. From earlier chapters you now realize that love is not unconditional. Relationships can and do change over time. Life can be unpredictable. If you know other couples that divorced, such as parents, siblings, or friends, you may want to discuss what you learned from watching them go through the process that will make it less likely that you will repeat the same mistakes.

Make a list of potentialities that you want to discuss with your partner. If you are planning on having children, talk about whether both of you will continue to work or if one of you wants to stay home to raise the kids. Should there be a recognition and consideration for the stay-at-home parent who is foregoing individual career opportunities and financial gains? What if one of you earns a master's degree in the course of your marriage and your partner supports you through that period? Should there be some consideration of that in your agreement? Clearly, there are a lot of things to consider. But I believe that if partners are given time and space to discuss and explore their needs, thoughts, and feelings, it can alleviate a lot of concern.

Setting down on paper what each of you will give up in the event that your marriage ends can serve as encouragement for working harder to keep your marriage healthy.

Money is not everything, but it is still a critical component in our lives. The bottom line to success in managing money in a marriage is communication, complete honesty, mutual responsibility, and shared goals. Establishing those priorities and getting the division of responsibility clear in advance can save you both from a lot of problems along the way.

POINTS TO REMEMBER

- Work together to create and respect your shared budget, and listen to each other when you have concerns, complaints, or fears about money.

- Agree on a spending limit for your joint budget, above which you will consult with each other.

- Recognize it is becoming more common for a woman to outearn her husband. This can be an area of contention and sensitivity when egos get involved.

- If you decide to have a stay-at-home parent, this decision should be revisited no less than once a year to determine if it still works for the family. The spouse who chooses to stay at home should make him or herself fully aware of the potential risks of doing so.

- Make sure you are fully informed about the amount of debt that each party brings to the relationship or that he or she is currently incurring.

- Avoid financial infidelity. Honesty and openness in financial matters serves to create and maintain trust in a long-term relationship. Financial secrets, once exposed, can put the foundation of your relationship at risk.

- Consider the potential upsides to having a prenup, especially when one or both of you come to the marriage with significant assets, debts, or when there are kids involved.

For more resources, go to:
www.DrAnneMalec.com

CHAPTER SEVEN:

The Case for Good Sex

A colleague of mine has a comic strip posted in her office that shows a man and woman sitting on a couch holding signs. The woman's sign says "no sex without love" and the man's says "no love without sex." It serves as a reminder that love and sex are mutually reinforcing and mean different things to different people. Sex often functions as a barometer for a relationship, in that if partners are struggling in their relationship, it manifests in their sexual intimacy, and if partners are struggling in their sexual relationship, it is often reflected in other areas of their marriage. At its best, sex is a means for creating and sustaining emotional and physical intimacy and connection. It provides an opportunity to give and receive needed physical pleasure while also providing many short- and long-term benefits for individual and relational well-being. At its worst, an unsatisfying sexual relationship can lead to loneliness, feelings of rejection or shame, and the end of a marriage. Sex is, therefore, an important component of healthy relationships.

Many married couples are interested in knowing where they fall on the sexual frequency scale. Researchers recently surveyed 70,000 individuals to assess the average sex life and found that 7.5 percent reported having sex daily, 40 percent had sex three to four times per week, 27 percent have sex a few times per month, 9 percent reported having sex once per month, 13 percent reported having sex rarely, and 4.5 percent never had sex.[31] However, the only crucial average of sexual frequency is the average you as a couple are happy with. Every couple and partner is different. Whether sexual intimacy occurs daily, once per week, once per month or less frequently, the important thing is that both parties are satisfied with the frequency. Do not judge yourselves on a "national average."

Sexual intimacy can and often does change over the course of a marriage and is not always indicative of a struggling relationship. Fluctuations in sexual desire and frequency are normal and should be expected. It does not mean you are with the wrong partner. Sexual frequency can change for many reasons unrelated to the quality of your relationship, including aging, physiological changes, illness, hormonal fluctuations, reduced desire, mental health struggles, and stress. Other sexual problems are caused by deterioration in the quality of a relationship and can be symptoms of poor marital communication, anger, and resentment; an unsatisfactory sex life can further corrode the perceived quality of a relationship. It is important for partners to grasp the benefits of a healthy sexual relationship and remain cognizant of the reinforcing relationship between sex and other aspects of a marriage, including intimacy and commitment.

PHYSICAL AND EMOTIONAL BENEFITS OF SEX

Sex is not just good for relationships; it is also good for *you*. Take a look at the health benefits of sex, of which there are a wide variety for both partners.

- Sex has a **positive impact on your immune system.** Those who regularly have sex have higher levels of the antibody immunoglobulin A or IgA, which protects you from colds and other infections.[32]

- **Sex has a positive impact on your overall fitness.** It lowers your blood pressure and burns about five calories per minute (four more calories per minute than watching TV), according to WebMD.[33]

- A good sex life is also **good for your heart.** Besides being a great way to raise your heart rate, sex helps to keep your estrogen and testosterone levels in balance, which also benefits the heart.

- **An enjoyable sex life lowers your stress level and improves your relationship,** not only by bringing you closer but because it wires your brain to associate pleasure with that person. Being close to your partner can reduce feelings of stress and anxiety with the release of the hormone oxytocin, which can lead to a stronger emotional connection. Sexual arousal releases a brain chemical that revs up your brain's pleasure and reward system, which leads to decreased levels of stress and anxiety.[34]

- The physical exercise **promotes better sleep.** After an orgasm, prolactin is released in your body, which is responsible for increased feelings of relaxation and sleepiness. Please note here that to experience the full benefit, sex requires that both partners achieve orgasm.[35]

- Sex also **improves women's bladder control,** because good sex provides a workout for your pelvic floor muscles, and orgasm causes contractions and strengthens those muscles.[36]

- **Having sex boosts libido.** Just like expending energy during exercise can lead to increased energy, frequent sex leads to desire for more frequent sex.[37]

CONSTRAINTS TO SEXUAL DESIRE

Given all the benefits, why would anyone say no to sex with his or her partner? Lack of sexual desire can be related to physical pain, the failure to achieve orgasm, marital unhappiness, anger, poor communication, lack of physical attraction, or resentment. A 2012 study by Murray and Milhausen found that heterosexual women's sexual desire decreased in direct correlation with the length of a relationship.[38] I would hypothesize that the same is likely true for men, and this is partially due to human nature. Habituation, the process of getting used to our partners, can lead to a decrease in desire and sexual frequency. Like any other activity, after engaging in it tens, hundreds, or thousands of times, sex can lose some of its newness, particularly if the couple engages in the same routines and behaviors prior to and during the act of intercourse. Sex may still be good, or maybe even great, but desire may lessen if there is no mystery and sex is too predictable.

It is also important to consider the nature of physical attraction and its relation to sexual desire. Remember how good you wanted to look for your partner when you began dating? Remember what it felt like to know your partner found you attractive? Ideally, partners will continue to prioritize health and fitness and maintain an interest in appearing attractive to each other. Not every partner needs a spouse with an athletic body type, but most partners desire a spouse who will make an effort to please them. This might mean wearing sexy lingerie every so often, maintaining a certain physique, or committing to a shaving regimen (remember, kissing with a beard can hurt). Society tends to emphasize the importance of women being sexually attractive to their partners (Victoria's Secret, for example), but less pressure is placed on men to be sexually attractive. I am not sure if there is a male equivalent to lingerie, but attention to hygiene, overall health and fitness, and remembering that foreplay starts long before you hit the bedroom is a good start!

Physical attraction continues to be an important component in a long-term sexual relationship, effort matters. It is a very difficult and sensitive issue to talk about between partners, but it is not uncommon for partners to lose interest in sex because the other has stopped exercising, gained weight, or stopped caring about his or her appearance. And it is rarely as superficial as desiring a physically attractive mate. For some partners, seeing you stop trying to maintain your physical appearance may communicate to your partner that he or she is no longer worth the effort.

There are several physiological factors unrelated to the marital relationship that may constrain sexual desire. According to the Mayo Clinic, the following diseases can lead to decreased desire: arthritis, cancer, diabetes, high blood pressure, coronary artery disease, and neurological diseases. Many medications can lessen desire, including some antidepressants and anti-seizure medications. Alcohol and drugs also lead to a diminished sex drive, as can simple fatigue.

Hormonal shifts in women can cause a loss of desire. The significant hormonal changes that occur during pregnancy, just after having a baby, and during breast-feeding, often put a damper on a couple's sex life—not to mention the exhaustion a new baby brings. Body image often suffers after childbirth, which can make a woman feel less desirable. And if women are nursing, sex with their partners can feel like just another claim on their time and bodies.

Performance anxiety can significantly influence a man's comfort level in the act of sex. If a man has suffered from erectile dysfunction (ED), there will likely be some anxiety around achieving and maintaining an erection. A woman needs to be extra sensitive with her partner if he has struggled with ED in the past or present. For men, much more so than women, sexual intimacy requires them to perform, so it is important not to put pressure on him and not to express disappointment if he has trouble with ED. The first step for dealing with ED is undergoing a thorough medical checkup, and there are therapies available to help (see www.DrAnneMalec.com).

Stress and mental health problems, such as depression, can negatively impact desire, as can poor body image or low self-esteem. A history of physical or sexual abuse can also lead to decreased desire for sex. Victims of sexual abuse are susceptible to flashbacks during sexual activity that are almost like re-traumatizations, so it is not unusual if they are inclined to shy away from intimacy. If this applies to you, please get help from a therapist, and do discuss your feelings with your partner so that he or she can understand what you are experiencing.

WORKING TOWARD A HAPPY SEX LIFE

How can you maintain sexual desire in your relationship? Leading sex and intimacy researcher Esther Perel speaks of maintaining desire by reconciling two fundamental human needs: "the need for security and predictability and the need for novelty, mystery, and the unexpected."[39] As monogamous partners, we value a spouse that we can trust and understand. As sexual beings, we crave mystery and are turned off by stagnation. Rather than pitting these basic human needs against each other, a satisfying sex life requires thought, creativity, and imagination. This does not mean you need to fantasize about sex with someone else in order to enjoy intimacy with your partner, but imagination plays a significant role in inspiring novelty within an established relationship. Imagine you and your partner are in a tropical location, be creative and try new acts of foreplay, and remember that it does not always need to be a physical act that gets you in the mood. Practice thinking of ways to introduce spontaneity and newness into your sex life.

There is a commonly held assumption that it is usually the woman who loses interest in sex—but this is not always the case. Both women and men can experience a loss of interest in sex. In my practice, the first thing I recommend to anyone experiencing sexual dissatisfaction or low sexual frequency is to get a thorough medical checkup, since sometimes loss of desire is related to a physical, medically treatable problem. In the absence of a health issue, we begin to talk about relationship issues. All relationship problems can lead to a loss of attraction and desire. Unresolved conflicts, undiscussed issues, lurking resentments—any of these can torpedo intimacy. Some of the common contributors include lack of connection, communication problems, and an underlying anger or frustration about some other aspect of your relationship.

Good sex requires that we allow ourselves to be vulnerable, to connect. If you feel that your partner is not listening to you or is not respectful or loving toward you, or if you feel taken for granted, these feelings might lead to a decreased desire for sex. Commonly a woman feels as though the only time her partner wants to touch her is when he wants sex. We all need physical expressions of love and affection on a daily basis; both men and women need and desire affection separate from sexual requests. When physical or intimate expression is confined to sexual inter- course, partners can feel neglected, pressured, and undesired. By expanding the definition of physical intimacy to include smaller acts of affection, like holding hands, real hugs that last for at least seven seconds, or kissing good night, both partners can feel safe and loved, two powerful prerequisites to sexual desire.

Poor communication between partners about sexual needs and preferences is also a common problem among couples with sexual dissatisfaction. Sex can be difficult or embarrassing to talk about, but your problems will not dissipate by simply ignoring them. I recognize that for many people, talking openly with a partner about your sexual likes and dislikes can feel awkward and uncomfortable. We live in a hyper-sexualized culture where the media inundates us with sexual images, but for some, the topic creates embarrassment or shame. The messages your parents sent, sexual education provided by academic institutions, community/ social expectations, and religious beliefs or training all impact one's openness to discussing sexual topics. Did your parents model effective communication about sexuality? Was sexuality ignored within your home? Did your religion create a sense of shame around sexual activity? For women in our culture, it may feel promiscuous and too aggressively sexual to openly talk with a partner about ways to enliven your sexual relationship. It is not unusual to feel uncomfortable with the topic, but it will benefit you and your relationship to learn how to communicate effec- tively about it.

Many couples come to me hoping to reignite the sexual spark in their relationship, to revive the passion that existed in the first year or two that the partners were together. Every couple wanting to reignite the spark has to be willing to put in the effort and set the stage for it to happen. This can be as simple as scheduling a time for sex. Some couples resist this planning piece, because it somehow seems "unsexy," not spontaneous enough, or even like a failure—but if you think back to when you were first dating, that was not exactly spontaneous either. You knew where you were going out for dinner. You knew what you were going to wear. You knew if your roommate was going to be home. And the anticipation that you would end your evening with sexual intimacy did not diminish the pleasure but likely improved it.

So try making a plan. If you have kids, plan for them to be out or asleep. Be aware that you and your partner may differ in when you are most open to sex. You may want sex at night when your partner is exhausted, and he or she may push for sex first thing in the morning, at a time when you typically snooze the alarm three times before opening your eyes. Rejection of sex due to exhaustion is rarely a reflection of your partner's feelings for you, so do not take it personally. Set the stage so you will not feel rejected, and talk about it: "When would you like to have sex?" Make it a regular thing, and enjoy looking forward to it.

Perceived rejection is one of the most common killers of sexual desire. If a man asks his wife to have sex, and she repeatedly turns him down, he often views her rejection as a rejection of him as a whole, not just sexually. This can cause him to feel that his wife is not interested in him, and ultimately he may stop asking altogether. He would like to be seen as a desirable man and capable of giving as well as receiving pleasure. **Your husband wants to know you desire him, just as you want to know he desires you.** A woman would certainly feel the same way if the situation were reversed, that is, if her partner frequently rejected her requests for sexual intimacy, she would feel rejected as a person. Nobody wants to feel like an unattractive, burdensome person. If you are the pursuer being repeatedly rejected, try something different, like asking your partner what turns him or her on. As the partner saying no, what is keeping you from saying yes? How can you set the stage to make it more likely that you will say yes? Figure it out, and if possible, share it with your partner.

Fostering desire means allowing the time for foreplay and making sure your partner understands your needs. It is not unusual for a woman to require more foreplay to become mentally engaged and physically aroused, so it is important to determine how much she needs and proceed accordingly! Think of foreplay as starting outside of the bedroom, and try viewing it as a function of how you treat your partner overall. The kinder you are to your partner in areas unrelated to sex, the more frequently you are likely to have sex and the better the sex is likely to be. As I said above, regular, daily expression of nonsexual affection is a big part of showing love for your partner and should never stop. Rushing through foreplay because you are physically ready for intercourse but your partner is not could derail the entire process, setting the stage for a one-sided sexual experience or mutual disappointment. Do not forget that kissing is the gateway to intimacy! (After all, when you first met, that is where it all began). Find your patience and become attuned to when your partner is ready.

For those who struggle to turn off their minds after a busy day, a frequent downside to our multitasking existence, you may benefit from becoming skilled at clearing your mind and learning to focus more on your body. Figure out what it takes for you to wind down and get in the mood, share this insight with your partner, and then do it. Gentle stretches, yoga poses, and meditation may be able to assist with quieting your mind and getting you in touch with your body. It is okay for you to ask your partner for help in achieving the right mindset. Back massages, help getting chores out of the way, and listening to music can ease one's mind, allowing space for desire to take root and blossom.

Be alert for the tendency to withhold sex as a punishment or bestow it as a reward. Although partially motivated by human nature, it is more often harmful to your relationship. It can be confusing, hurtful, and damaging to your partner's trust and desire. Men who struggle with emotional expression often rely on sex to feel emotionally connected to a woman. It is not just about physical release but about vulnerability and fostering an emotional and romantic connection with his partner. Sex should be for the benefit of both of you; by denying your partner, you are also denying yourself. Rewarding your partner with sex sends the message that you feel only one of you benefits from sex. I cannot help but find it similar to giving a dog a treat for rolling over on command. Gratitude and appreciation for certain behaviors or tasks should be separate from sexual intimacy, and sex should not be used as one-sided currency.

If you find yourself frequently denying sex to your partner due to feelings of resentment, anger, or unresolved conflict, tell him or her what is keeping you from desiring physical intimacy. Frequent denials lead to fewer attempts at initiating, which lead to both emotional and physical disconnection and a weak marital foundation. In order for an issue to be resolved, it must be communicated.

Some couples may have difficulty with sexual intimacy or in frequency because the woman does not have an orgasm during intercourse. This can make her feel both unsatisfied and less interested in sex. Why do women orgasm less frequently during sex than men? The Mayo Clinic states that the female "sexual response involves a complex interaction of physiology, emotions, experiences, beliefs, lifestyles, and relationships. Disruption of any of these components can affect sexual drive, arousal, or satisfaction."[40] It is easier for women to get distracted during sexual interactions, and unlike men, they receive conflicting cultural messages about fully expressing their sexuality. Whatever the cause, if a woman is not having an orgasm, she is most likely not going to want to have sex, and this negatively affects both parties. Women who think, "Let's just get this over with," are often not having orgasms—and this attitude can kill the mood. Your partner can usually tell when you are having obligatory sex.

It is of critical importance to the relationship that both parties reach climax (at least most of the time), whether in intercourse or foreplay. The pleasure you receive from your orgasm is often equal to or surpassed by the pleasure felt from gifting an orgasm to your partner. That is why foreplay is important in getting a woman aroused, because women (as well as men) are more likely to engage in behaviors that feel good than in those that do not. It is not just the woman's issue. Men enjoy sex more when they know their partners are sexually satisfied. If a woman denies her need for sexual satisfaction, if she feels no physical benefit from intercourse, she may eventually lose interest altogether, begin engaging in obligatory sex, and lose this vital connection to her partner.

Sometimes, of course, there are more serious issues behind the loss of desire, such as a breach of trust in the relationship, like infidelity. In this situation, not only is there a sense of rejection and unattractiveness, resulting in emotional pain, but an affair also sparks worry about sexually transmitted diseases. People who have been hurt by a partner through infidelity can suffer artificial flashbacks where even thoughts of sex trigger visions of one's partner with the affair partner. Sexually motivated affairs often have many warning signs, including an inappropriate attraction for another person, secretly communicating or meeting with another person in a way that your partner would not approve of, and having sexual fantasies about a specific person that you know. Before acting on these urges, try to understand what is missing in your marriage and sex life with your spouse. See if you can talk to your partner about it, and seek outside assistance in having this conversation before committing a physical act of betrayal. As I will talk more about in chapter 10, infidelity is traumatizing, and it is a hard thing for couples to overcome alone. If you recently experienced an affair, please seek help from a therapist to evaluate the future of your relationship.

BALANCING PARENTHOOD WITH A HEALTHY SEX LIFE

I previously discussed the issues that new moms can have with sex due to changes in hormones, exhaustion, and body image problems—but another issue I would like to mention is the frequency of postpartum depression (PPD) and its relationship to sex. It is estimated that symptoms of PPD occur in approximately 8–19 percent of mothers and 4 percent of fathers during the child's first year of life.[41] PPD can also occur in women who miscarry or give birth to stillborn children. PPD affects approximately 900,000 couples each year.[42] Like depression, PPD can inhibit sexual desire and lead to disconnection between partners.

You may be at risk of PPD if you experience the following:

- Trouble sleeping when your baby sleeps (more than the lack of sleep new moms usually get)

- Feeling numb or disconnected from your baby

- Having scary or negative thoughts about the baby, like thinking someone will take your baby away or hurt your baby

- Worrying that you will hurt the baby

- Feeling guilty about not being a good mom or ashamed that you cannot care for your baby[43]

Another issue that can affect sexual desire and intimacy in a marriage post-childbirth, is men reacting negatively to being in the delivery room to watch the birth of their child. For some men, observing the act of birth can be quite traumatizing. Men are very visual creatures, for better or worse. Although the idea of being together for the birth may initially sound romantic, a couple might want to think very hard about what the spouse is exposed to in the delivery room. In watching childbirth, the mystery, the sensuality of sex, and the female's sexual organs can become something akin to "plumbing." Some men have difficulty erasing this image from their minds. Psychologist Shoshana Bennett shares that the delivery room experience can be unexpected and even traumatic for some partners due to the process of "watching another human being emerge from the part once considered purely for sexual pleasure."[44]

Of course, this reaction does not occur with all men, or even most men, but it does happen. It is not a frequently discussed topic, because it feels controversial, and men probably feel like jerks in even mentioning it. After a woman goes through nine months of pregnancy and an intense delivery, it can feel inconsiderate and melodramatic for husbands to complain, let alone feel traumatized, about *their* experience. That is why discussing fears and expectations throughout the pregnancy can help a couple prepare and maintain boundaries around the delivery process. The husband should be a full partner in this final leg of pregnancy but, as a couple, try to figure out beforehand how much he wants to see and how much she wants him to see.

Kids, whether they are infants, toddlers, or school-age, create obstacles to intimacy. You now have much less time to devote solely to your relationship because of your job as parents, and viewing sex as a chore rather than a time of connection reduces the likelihood that it will happen. It is normal for partners to shift their sexual frequency and intimacy patterns after having children, but focusing on your children to the exclusion of your relationship introduces new risks to your sex life. Your marriage is *not* self-sustaining: it needs the two of you to keep moving the ball down the field. Prioritize your couple relationship, make time for your sexual intimacy needs, and find a healthy balance between couple time and parent time. You will not regret making your relationship the priority, and your kids will benefit from being raised by happy and loving parents.

Sexuality does not end because of advancing age. It is a necessary and healthy part of a happy marriage, the most intimate form of loving communication you can share. If for some reason that part of your marriage is not working for both of you, take whatever steps are necessary to get back on track, and rediscover your lover.

=== **POINTS TO REMEMBER** ===

- Regular, mutually satisfying sex enhances your marriage and your health.

- Hormonal shifts in either partner can impact sexual desire and performance, as can health issues or drug/alcohol abuse. If you are having problems, your first stop should be your doctor's office.

- Rejecting your partner too often can lead him or her to feel undesirable and ultimately to stop seeking intimacy.

- Other desire-killers include traumatic memories, resentment, or breaches of trust, like infidelity. Communicate your feelings to your partner, and if necessary, seek help from a qualified therapist.

- Needing more time to get aroused does not mean your female partner is not attracted to you. Female sexual arousal and desire can be more complex than men's. It is important to prioritize getting the woman mentally engaged for intimacy.

- Men can be traumatized by seeing their wives give birth, so if your husband has any hesitance about watching the actual delivery, do not push the issue.

- The tasks of parenthood can leave you feeling exhausted and without enough time in the day—two prime risk factors for losing sexual intimacy. Talk with your partner about ways you can still prioritize your sexual relationship, because it benefits both of you.

For more resources, go to:

www.DrAnneMalec.com

CHAPTER EIGHT:

Married While Parenting

In any relationship, kids are a game changer. Whether biological, adopted, or step-offspring, children add complexity to marriage. This chapter discusses the challenge inherent in staying emotionally and physically connected after children join your marriage. I do not include parenting advice, but focus on describing how to prioritize your relationship while simultaneously caring for and raising children.

Modern parents often feel added pressure to be hyper-focused on their children. This pressure can come as a reaction to the parenting they received (trying to mimic or parent oppositely) or be a means to assuage the guilt felt by working parents. Where our parents may have simply let us play outside, today's parent must arrange for play dates, classes, and make the large time and financial commitment to have children participate in organized sports. Today's society also encourages parents to involve their children in these activities at younger ages than in the past. Peer pressure and edicts that such efforts are necessary to give kids the best possible start in life trap modern parents in having little time to devote to themselves or their marriages.

Concurrent with the increase in parenting demands is the growing trend of dual-career families. The increased pressure leaves many parents feeling guilty about not spending enough or the right kind of time with their children. Working mothers feel an added burden to perform well at work and also satisfy modern parenting standards. This can come at the cost of personal and relational well-being.

THE CHALLENGES OF TRANSITIONING FROM 2 TO 3

Realistic expectations about how kids change a marriage help couples minimize the common struggle of transitioning to parenthood. The first step in setting yourselves up to be successful is accepting that having children will be a game changer for each of you and for your relationship.

Following the birth of a child, your marriage abruptly goes from being the number-one priority—as it was when you were dating and newly married—to number two as each partner faces the responsibility and hard work of caring for a newborn. Both parents may feel less special to their mate and lose a degree of autonomy, independence, and freedom of action. New parents also frequently experience insecurity about their parenting abilities, underscoring the pull to prioritize the parenting relationship.

Being a new parent takes an adjustment, and it often affects each couple and partner differently. Unfortunately, the new family member will not consider your needs at all. He or she will wake you frequently, at times be inconsolable, make non-stop messes, take no account of your schedule, occasionally make you miss work, and generally leave you exhausted, cranky, and short-tempered toward a spouse that is going through the exact same thing! Having too little time and energy for all of your responsibilities will naturally make you worry about how well you are doing as a parent, as a partner, and as an employee. Young children require great gobs of time and significant amounts of attention, love, nurturing, and financial support. It is like having another full-time job—but working for a 'boss' that does not care about excuses or honor vacation days.

It is easy to see why adding children detracts from the time, attention, and energy that partners have for each other. This is normal. It does not mean you are a bad parent or a bad partner. The transition to parenthood requires mutual flexibility and an active plan to meet all of one's responsibilities. This plan must start with the active involvement of both parents.

With the arrival of a newborn, fathers often feel that they are relegated to a distant second place in their wives' attention. Fathers may also feel like they are in second place with the new baby because they cannot naturally provide the most basic need —food. New dads must realize and accept this is the new, but hopefully temporary, reality. New moms can help their partners understand that the dislocation is a temporary necessity to keep the family functioning. View yourselves as a team with the joint goal of smoothing the transition from the life of a couple to a family. And, like any team, each player has responsibilities. Regularly discuss those responsibilities and check in with your partner about any needs that are not being met.

Advice for Those in the Trenches of New Parenthood:

- The sleepless nights might seem interminable, but this period of your life is temporary. It is the price of admission to being a parent.

- Chronic sleep deprivation will create tension, frustration, and short tempers, so try not to hold a snarky comment made in the middle of the night against your partner.

- Being tired can lead to forgetfulness or cognitive slowness. Things may need to be repeated more than once.

- Try to not insult or criticize a partner whose parenting style is different than yours. Doing something differently does not mean it is wrong, and all new parents learn as they go. To achieve full partner participation, you must be willing to let your partner do it his or her way.

- Agree to dedicate time and resources to keeping the connection between the two of you healthy and loving. Parenting can take over your lives if you do not make date night a priority.

- Your individual emotional lives can function without attention for a little while, but do not let this become your permanent way of life. Make time to check in with each other and allow yourselves the opportunity for self-care.

- When you need help from your partner, ask for it. You are sharing in this new, great adventure.

- Set up a Parent-On-Duty system whereby you take turns taking full responsibility for all parenting duties. This allows for each of you to have time off to focus on non-parenting aspects of your lives.

- New parents also need the support and understanding of friends and family. Create schedules where you each get a girls' or guys' night out. Regardless of how great a relationship, none of us have all of our emotional needs met by our partners.

- Learn to communicate without creating more stress. If one parent is struggling with the child's behavior, asking "Can I help?" might be more productive than asking, "What is going on here?" Figure out a language that works for both of you.

- New moms often miss their social work environment after going on maternity leave and feel like they have less to contribute to daily conversation. They need their partners to want to hear about how they spend their day, even if it is just a report on the frequency of the baby's poops.

- Life will run more smoothly by coming to an agreement in advance on things like: Whose turn will it be tonight to get up with the baby? How do you share diaper changes? If the baby is not ill or in need but just fussy, will you let the baby "cry it out" or will one of you go to soothe the baby?

Initial Child-Care Decisions

During the pregnancy, many couples begin to discuss how they want to provide care for the child. Every couple has different needs, desires, and hopes for their new family, and having a practical discussion about how to handle this time when your child is most dependent upon you can save your relationship from a lot of stress later on.

Predicting how we will feel after a life-changing event is difficult. Determining how each of you will feel about specific child-care arrangements before the birth of a child is challenging and may fluctuate. There will be a host of unknowns and some misplaced assumptions. However, making plans in advance is a helpful way to practice communicating about parental matters, even if you change your mind after the baby is born. Nothing needs to be set in stone in the planning stage. What is important is learning the process of communicating and remaining flexible, open, and willing to compromise.

If you feel that it is best for one of you to stay at home, it may be beneficial to do so for a trial period to be sure that it is a workable solution. Being your child's full-time caregiver can be enriching, emotionally rewarding, and soul satisfying, but there are also tradeoffs if you are used to working in a professional office environment and being financially independent. If the two of you agree that one parent will stay home with your child, that decision should be revisited every year or so, perhaps close to your child's birthday. Is this care-giving structure still working? How is it not working? How can we make it work better? Does the at-home parent feel too isolated, anxious, frustrated, or mildly depressed about being out of the workforce? Does the working spouse feel overwhelming financial pressure to solely provide for the family? Just because it seemed best for your family at one point does not mean you are both stuck in this dynamic for the next 18 years. Maintain an open dialogue about your expectations and hopes for your family structure.

Mom at Work

After returning to work from maternity leave, new moms may initially feel as though they are underperforming at both home and work. Adding the role of mother on top of the previous roles of employee and wife is emotionally trying and exhausting. To help ease the transition, new moms need their partners to be supportive and considerate of any guilt, fear, or anxiety in leaving the child with a caregiver. It is typical to feel emotionally vulnerable and torn about handing your child over to a child care provider, particularly for new parents who were raised by a stay-at-home mother. It is normal for a new mom to experience contradictory emotions about returning to work, and this uncertainty can persist well after the decision is implemented. She may very much enjoy working, but she may also feel tremendous guilt about leaving her child. Her spouse should not dismiss or minimize such feelings, even if they appear contradictory. Providing emotional support will cultivate intimacy within your relationship and may shorten both the time and severity of any feelings of guilt.

What Your Marriage Needs

A frequent refrain of new parents is "We don't have time for date nights," or "We can't afford date nights because when you add the cost of a babysitter to dinner and a movie...." If you already struggle to find 20 minutes to sit down for a daily check-in, you may easily find reasons for why you cannot afford a weekly date night. But it is important to create couple time.

I understand how partners can feel so worn out from handling both a career and parenting that they do not want to have to do anything else. But there are many things in life besides children that require consistent care and nurturing, and a relationship is certainly one of them. Saying you cannot find time for your relationship is neglectful and hurtful to your partner and yourself. Nurturing your marriage must remain a priority. Scheduling a date night might feel like just one more thing that needs to be done, but all couples I have worked with report being happy that they made it happen and many wonder why they ever stopped. You may even find yourself happily anticipating the day as the week progresses (I know I do).

Get creative with scheduling couple time: meet for lunch during the week; arrange your child care provider to stay later one night a week and meet for dinner after work; meet in the family room at 9:00 p.m.; plan an at-home dinner date; or purchase tickets for plays, orchestras, concerts, sporting events, wine tastings, or other events. There are so many options! Take turns planning events away from home as well as in-home dates. Start doing it, and soon enough it will become a wonderful, healthy habit.

There is significant danger in not staying close as romantic partners while co-parenting. If you fail to make routine deposits to your relationship "retirement account", you may find yourself "broke" when your children leave home. Children want healthy, loving parents; parents that love not just them but each other as well. We all need love. You make efforts to ensure your children feel loved, and your mate deserves the same consideration.

Her Needs and His Needs

Along with your parental and relational responsibilities, you also need to care for yourself. Employed women can feel so guilty for not being able to spend more time with their children that they prioritize all of their at-home time to be focused on their children. Mothers may do so at the expense of their partner and themselves. Sometimes women have to be convinced that it is okay, even healthy, to engage in self-care; that is, to exercise, go out with friends, read a book, or sleep late. The painful irony is that in an effort to be the best parent, to create a home life in which your children feel loved, nurtured, and safe, you may lose your sense of self. If you are not happy with yourself, you are likely also unhappy in your relationship, and your partner will notice. Discuss ways you can help each other find time to care for yourselves.

It is not unusual for a new father to feel overwhelmed by the increased economic burden of providing for the new family unit. At least temporarily, you go from being a two-income couple to being a one-income-family of three. Depending upon child-care arrangements, this may be a long-term change in your family dynamic. This prospect creates real pressure for new dads, and tension may develop between two exhausted and overwhelmed partners. New dads may be sensitive to their partners expecting them to significantly share in child care if their partners fail to empathize with the stressors of being the sole provider. Exacerbated by exhaustion, conflict can easily erupt if both partners feel underappreciated and like they are not doing good enough in their multiple roles of spouse, parent, and provider.

There is little I can offer to soften the reality of this situation, but know that mutual empathy, appreciation, understanding, and expressions of affection can help smooth the way. Try to find the humor in all the new baby craziness, and bond over the exhaustion of "living the dream" of new parenthood.

SHARING THE LOAD

In marriages with kids, one of the biggest recurring conflicts develops around who does what. In couple sessions, I frequently hear resentment expressed about the unfair division of household and parenting responsibilities. Even when both partners are in the workforce, the majority of housework and child care can too frequently fall on the wife's shoulders. Related research on hours worked inside and outside the home provides interesting findings.

A research report published in 2011 reports that *on average* married women and men work an almost equal number of hours per week, with the breakdown shown on the following page:[45]

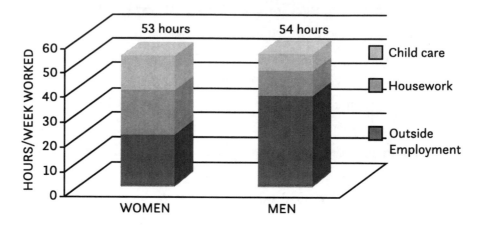

While the results show the average woman (with children under 18) works 21 hours per week outside the home, this average includes both women who don't work at all outside the home and those who do. The question becomes: what level of outside employment justifies one partner being responsible for spending twice as much time on housework and child care? If a woman is working 30-40 hours per week outside of the home, is it fair to ask that she put in an additional 30 hours per week toward home and child care? As more mothers choose to work full-time, this has become a major issue in modern marriages. Sometimes the added income allows parents to hire outside assistance to lighten the load on the couple. Family members, daycare, a nanny, or a weekly housekeeper can ease the burden on busy parents. For the remaining tasks, equitable sharing of home and child-care responsibilities creates marital harmony and satisfaction.

If one partner is earning substantially more than the other and is required to work long hours outside the home to earn this salary, this partner logically will perform less of the in-home work. Nonetheless, the "outside" partner will still likely be responsible for certain home or child care tasks and needs to show a willingness to do his or her fair share. When there is an imbalance in division of labor, partners must actively demonstrate an appreciation for their spouses' contributions, whether in child care, housework, or outside employment.

Sharing housework ranks third, after faithfulness and a happy sexual relationship, as the most important factor in determining marital satisfaction.[46] When men are perceived to do a fair share of household chores, couples report fewer conflicts, wives are happier and have lower rates of depression, and marriages have a lower rate of divorce.[47] Additionally, couples that share housework equally have more sex than couples who do not.[48] There is no magic equation to deem an equitable sharing arrangement for your marriage, and it is through continued discussion and trial and error that you and your partner must find and adjust your parameters. Your needs and expectations will change as your children age and partners exit or re-enter the workforce, so develop a routine with checks and balances to ensure a fair approach.

Start by talking about it with your partner—establish fair expectations, and plan how you can execute this together. Creating a spreadsheet of who does what and when can be effective in generating the sense that there is a fair split and ensures you are each aware of your responsibilities. Include everything you can think of that needs to be done to make your lives, your kids' lives, and your household run smoothly. You would not think twice about creating such a spreadsheet at work, so do the same at home. To see some ideas about what should be included, you can find a sample at www.DrAnneMalec.com.

As mentioned earlier in this book, if you want your partner to help you, ask for it! Be specific about what you want or need and when you would like it completed. Do not expect your partner to read your mind. Women may wonder "Why can't he see what needs being done?" The answer is because he is not looking through your eyes. That said, a man should not wait to be asked for help. When it comes to parenting the children, helping with dinner, or cleaning up a mess, a father is not there to serve as an assistant. He is an equal partner.

As an equal partner, a woman needs to accept and expect that her husband may parent differently (and different does not automatically mean wrong). If you want him to be a full partner in parenting, treat him like one. A child will not be permanently scarred by going to a fast food restaurant for lunch once in a while or from watching a little extra TV while a parent is trying to finish a report. Limit your criticisms and corrections, and remember that you must pick your battles to avoid damaging your marriage. If men are constantly criticized, they will back away and be less likely to fully engage.

The same goes for helping with housework. If a woman wants a genuinely fair division of household labor with a fully engaged partner, she needs to ease up on the specifics of how she wants things done. You married an intelligent, competent, nurturing, and caring person. If you are going to be critical and judgmental of a husband's approach to parenting or housework, he is going to withdraw and hesitate about reentering the fray. Let him do it his way, or calmly explain why you would like something to be done differently. For tasks that you need to be done in a specific way, it may be easier to do them yourself than to be frustrated by your partner's attempts. Remember, all of us are more likely to repeat behaviors for which we are positively rewarded. Be better at telling your partner the things he or she does correctly than in criticizing the things you would do differently. Thanks and appreciation go a long way.

The need for shared parenting responsibilities includes disciplinary actions. Some parents take to this role more easily than others. However, you want to avoid this job falling to one parent, as no one wants to feel like the "bad guy" all the time. Children require consistent structure, rules, and consequences; teaching your kids the rules that will allow them to live as responsible adults is a shared obligation of parenting.

BLENDED FAMILIES

Blended families, where one or both partners bring children from a prior relationship into the marriage, are increasingly common. When I married my husband, I chose to become part of a blended family. I became a stepparent in addition to becoming a wife. Because every blended family is different in its structure and make-up of members, locating resources that spoke specifically to my new family was a challenge. I imagine readers in blended families may feel the same way. As for me, I ultimately used a trial-and-error approach. And I still do.

Real blended families are not like the Brady Bunch, where newly joined family members seamlessly forge loving and playful bonds while never mentioning or spending time with the other biological parent. Blended families face unique challenges in maintaining marital harmony. The needs of the intimate relationship need to be balanced with those of the children. Blended families require significant organizational adjustments for all family members, and it can be difficult for partners to accept the gradual process necessary to establish a cohesive relational and family unit.

Manage Expectations

When creating a blended family, managing your expectations will decrease the odds of being disappointed. Discuss your ideas for how the transition will go, and set a reasonable bar for how you, your spouse, your kids, and your former spouse(s) will respond to the new arrangement. Organization, frequent communication, and shared schedules are of vital importance in establishing and maintaining a blended family. Expect and plan for a slow transition into this "new normal." Discuss your goals frequently, and determine consistent house rules so that all the children live by the same rules and expectations. Above all, be patient and flexible with your partner's needs and concerns, and use your daily and weekly check-ins to stay connected and organized.

Too frequently, partners imagine that because they love each other, their children will jump on board and will also love this new partner as a stepparent. In reality, children are often confused and have contradictory emotions about the new family setup. New couples may fail to give due consideration to the effect on their children of:

- feeling disloyal to the other birth parent by embracing a new stepparent;

- sharing a bedroom with a new stepsibling;

- feeling as though there are different rules for different kids (curfews, allowances, accepted behaviors);

- having to adjust to *another* living arrangement they had no say in;

- being "forced" to spend time with people they do not know or possibly like very much;

- having to share their parent with a new stepparent or step-siblings.

It can get complicated, fast. Understanding the struggles and complexities of what the children are dealing with can help to manage frustration and to foster empathy with their experience.

Parents may have to face the fact that their kids would rather stay at the other biological parent's house because it is less complicated than coming to the house with the new stepparent and stepsiblings that they had no voice in choosing. Giving your kids an appropriate voice in the process will go a long way toward easing the transition. Having low expectations does not mean that you willingly tolerate poor behavior or hostility from your children during this period, but seeing the situation from their perspective can go a long way to mitigating any disappointment should things not happen according to plan.

It is up to the new couple to develop strategies for handling the transition to a blended family. Each parent should be responsible for managing his or her children's schedules, providing discipline, and communicating with the ex-partner about any parenting issues. You should expect that it is going to be a rocky ride, and you can be pleasantly surprised if it is not. The kids did not get a vote in this, and they very well may dislike the stepparent or stepsiblings. There can be personality conflicts, they may have been holding out hope that their parents would get back together, or they may not like the stepparent because he or she was an affair partner during the parents' marriage. Listen to your children's concerns, empathize with them, but always convey compassion for the new spouse and hope for the new family.

Spouses should also be aware of their sensitivities regarding the new family; you or your partner will probably feel guilty about having put your children through a divorce, so you may be highly sensitive to how the new partner treats your kids. You may have different expectations or rules around behavior, discipline, consequences, curfews, and spending money. Compounding the problem is that your kids keep track of inconsistencies and see who is getting treated differently. Be aware of your sensitivities and emotional triggers, and accept that your new family is a work in progress.

Communications with Former Spouses

The manner and frequency with which you communicate with a former spouse can have a significant influence on how you transition into your new family. Some relationships with exes run smoother than others. Ideally, former spouses communicate respectfully, keeping in mind the best interests of the children, and maintain boundaries around any new romantic relationships. However, in reality, the incompatibility that led to divorce may complicate the coparenting relationship.

Having to coparent with an ex-spouse who continues to harbor resentment and anger about the divorce can be emotionally painful. The discord between exes can bleed into the current marital relationship in the form of frustration, bad moods, distraction, or continued arguments and conflict. It is hard to feel emotionally connected with a partner when it feels like his or her former spouse continues to take up a lot of negative emotional space. If you have an ex-spouse who continues to press your buttons, annoys you, or creates other negative feelings, it is important for you to figure out a way to process these feelings as they arise. You may want to consider consulting with a therapist or engaging in some of the self-soothing techniques I describe in chapter 2: meditating, exercising, taking a walk, journaling, completing a task, and so on.

It will benefit your current relationship if you can minimize the conflict with a former partner. It is not easy to be respectful or uphold a joint parenting agreement when your ex-spouse is not doing the same. But you will probably feel better about yourself if you try. If possible, work with a former partner to establish joint rules of behavior for your children to be followed in both homes. Communicate as often as necessary, and try not to use your children as messengers.

If you get along well with a former partner and have been able to divorce and coparent amicably (which is very beneficial for your children), your new partner may be sensitive to or feel threatened by any perceived emotional closeness with your ex. After all, at one point in time you felt the same about your ex as you do about your current partner. This does not mean that your relationship with your ex is necessarily inappropriate or that your new spouse is being irrational. Any marriage requires adaptation and flexibility, and a major challenge with the formation of blended families is balancing the needs of your role as spouse with those as parent. Do what you can to maintain respectful boundaries and ensure that your communication with your ex centers on the needs of your children.

Nurture Your Romance

Due to the challenges of balancing parental and relational responsibilities, the blended family dynamic requires extra effort toward maintaining sufficient kid-free time. Making time for just the two of you is critical to the success of your relationship. Without proper attention, the new relationship can fall down the priority list amongst everything else the new couple faces: smoothing the transition for the children, creating a blended home, trying to grow comfortable with the role of stepparent, etc. It is not unusual for partners to be hyper-focused on the adjustment of their respective children, but the new spouse is probably having some difficulty adapting to the new family as well. There are a lot of balls in the air, and some may drop from time to time. Just make sure to pick them back up. Make it through the tough days by maintaining healthy, open, and honest communication about any struggles or difficulties either of you encounter in your transition to blended family status. Bonding over a shared struggle will go a long way toward sustaining your emotional intimacy.

The challenges of blended families are different and more complex than the challenges facing partners in a first marriage. As suggested in earlier chapters, it is important to take every opportunity to just be together with your new partner—to take time to communicate, commiserate, bond, and share the bad with the good. Make it a point to prioritize dates, whether over coffee, lunch, dinner, or during a walk together. Schedule the time for daily and weekly check-ins, budget discussions, and so on. If possible, arrange parenting schedules with your ex-spouse that allow you to have sufficient nonparenting, partner-focused time. Try to get away by yourselves at least twice a year. Be sure to tell your partner when you need him or her to listen or to help you problem-solve. Be mindful of not reacting too harshly when your partner struggles with or criticizes the words or actions of your offspring. Seek support, and if needed, contact a couple and family therapist for help.

To maintain a healthy and satisfying marriage, it is essential to keep the lines of communication open—between you and your spouse and you and your kids. Knowing in advance that it is likely to be tough and keeping your expectations dialed down can go a long way toward making sure that your relationship does not fall apart under the stress.

POINTS TO REMEMBER

- Parents need to agree on appropriate rules for parenting and revisit them regularly—ones that reflect their thoughts and values.

- Children do best in a family where both parents have equal involvement in their upbringing.

- Becoming a parent does not negate your intimate relationship as a priority. Remember to designate sufficient couple time to stay connected with your partner.

- Forming a blended family is a long-term process, and it is reasonable to expect some pushback from the children, who have had no voice in your choice to marry. Be patient, and try to see it through their eyes.

For more resources, go to:
www.DrAnneMalec.com

CHAPTER NINE:

Slippery Slopes

Romantic partners enter slippery slopes through bad relationship habits that go unacknowledged or unaddressed. Common culprits include resentment, dismissiveness, overuse or addiction to substances or other harmful behaviors, emotional disconnection leading to a lack of physical intimacy, ineffective communication habits, and inappropriate extramarital relationships. What these behaviors have in common is that they all take a toll on a marriage, and they all reflect a partner putting other interests ahead of his or her spouse instead of facing the issues that currently exist in the marriage.

Unaddressed issues frequently fester beneath one or both partners' awareness until both partners find themselves too far apart for reconciliation without outside assistance. It is often easier to eliminate problematic behavior early on than it is to recover from the long-term consequences of problematic behavior. The tricky part is to be willing to hear your partner's request for change when it is first brought to your attention.

RESENTMENT

Dismissiveness leads to resentment, and resentment damages relationships, sometimes permanently. What does dismissiveness look like? Dismissiveness occurs when your partner shares his or her feelings and thoughts with you, and instead of listening, you actively disregard the comments and fail to empathize with what your partner has to say. Dismissiveness is immediately rolling your eyes when you hear something you dislike, giving in to your knee-jerk reaction instead of attempting to understand your partner's perspective. The message is: "I cannot believe you are (still) talking about this!" or "You have no right to (insert the comment or question your partner said here)" or "Why are you wasting my time with this?" You get my point. Dismissiveness is the equivalent of flipping your partner the bird. It is treating your partner with contempt.

How does such deep-seated resentment develop? While one party may not feel that he or she has committed any relationship sin, the other partner may feel that he or she has lived with a steady diet of not being heard, respected, looked at, or given affection. Such partners do not feel appreciated or supported; in general, they do not feel like their emotional well-being is taken into consideration by their partner. Not doing your fair share; not living within an agreed budget; being dishonest, passive-aggressive, or defensive; frequent yelling—all of these roads lead to resentment.

Resentment does not develop overnight. It is pernicious in that its power grows in cumulative increments. Resentment is like a minor wound that is left to fester for too long. Instead of healing, as it would if treated immediately, the wound becomes infected due to gross neglect or a series of ineffectual short-term fixes. It can be difficult to pin down where and when the resentment developed because of the systemic nature of relationships; it is hard to know who or what started the process. Try to avoid finger-pointing and blame, as these are only time wasters and will only exacerbate the problem. Instead, focus on what needs to change in order for resentment to be replaced by connection and empathy.

Perhaps you have experienced a situation like this in your relationship: you feel as though your partner treats you disrespectfully, and so you respond in one of these ways:

1. Point out what your partner said or did that hurt your feelings, and ask him or her to stop it.

2. Ask your partner what is upsetting him or her and why you are being treated in this way.

3. Ignore it (initially), and hope it stops.

4. Treat your partner disrespectfully in retaliation.

Options 1 and 2 are preferable for directly addressing perceived disrespect, but for the conflict-avoidant person, these options may seem too risky, as these strategies may open up your relationship to even more conflict. If your default approach is to ignore it or strike back with more disrespect, recognize that as a long-term strategy, these two options are dead-ends. As partners in relationships, few of us are willing to tolerate disrespect or dismissiveness without firing back in some way; either with dismissiveness of our own or through passive aggression. Partners strike back to maintain relational balance and to send the message that the treatment is unacceptable. But meeting disrespect with more disrespect leads to emotional escalation and ugliness and rarely allows your partner to understand that he or she treated you poorly. The best strategy to address the situation is to confront the disrespect directly before the harmful pattern takes hold of your relationship.

I recognize that some topics between partners are tiresome, boring, or conflict-ridden, and from time to time we are all susceptible to acting dismissively or disrespectfully—particularly when we are tired or stressed. But be mindful that dismissiveness does not become your go-to response. Your partner feels the disdain it shows. It wears on the relationship and chips away at the foundation of your love and commitment.

Resisting Resentment

If a spouse feels that his or her partner is frequently dismissive and recognizes that it is damaging the relationship, ideally that spouse will bring these feelings to the partner's attention. However, frequently what happens is that the dismissed partner gets angry and resentful and eventually chooses to emotionally check out of the relationship. It may not feel like it, but becoming resentful without telling your partner is a choice. Before resentment becomes the norm, try to find that vulnerable place in yourself and talk honestly about how your partner hurt you or about other concerning behaviors. Be specific about the action or words that create your upset feelings. This can feel challenging, especially if your partner acts defensively and you have had little success in resolving past conflicts. You may feel that it is easier to ignore your feelings rather than risk your partner becoming upset, making you feel even more distant and hurt. But choosing to live with ongoing resentment and denying your needs for kindness, respect, and caring can damage your self-esteem and your relationship.

Resentment can be stopped in its tracks if you approach your partner and say, "I need to talk about this, and I need you to really hear me: I am worried about your spending, drinking, Internet use, poor diet..." or "I am angry and upset by your unwillingness to talk to me about our problems, your never being willing to finish a difficult conversation, your use of the silent treatment..." Without directly addressing resentment, one of two things usually happens: a spouse emotionally shuts down and becomes disengaged, or the resentment comes out as explosive anger during a fight. Resentment simmers quietly in the background unless and until it is faced.

Choose to fight resentment by honestly confronting a problem that is affecting your relationship. You show respect for yourself and your relationship by making time to talk and openly communicate about conflicts or points of difference that need to be heard. Diminish resentment by creating a safe emotional space and a healthy problem-resolution approach. Become skilled at listening and addressing the problems or conflicts that arise between you. Work together to problem-solve. It is not easy, but it is a necessary skill that can be acquired with due practice and is a marriage saver.

Addressing Resentment with Your Partner

Here are a few easy ways to start this type of conversation:

- "I would like to talk about _____ (fill in the blank). I'm feeling very disconnected from you, and it's making me feel sad and scared. I think it stems from when you said..."

- "I'm angry, and I don't want to be, so I need to talk about..."

- "I've tried to communicate about this issue before but would like to try again. Is there a good time to talk later today or tomorrow?"

- "I love you and want to stay close to you, so I want to say that I am feeling upset about..."

- "I am feeling distant or isolated from you; can we find time to connect later?"

- "When I feel like you ignore me, ridicule me, or treat me disrespectfully, I grow angry and resentful, and it pushes me away from you. It most frequently happens when _____. Please stop treating me this way."

Listening to Your Partner's Resentment

When your partner attempts to talk to you about his or her resentment, it is easy to become defensive if you feel attacked or misinterpreted. Remember that having a different perspective does not make either of you right or wrong, and it is important to be an active listener to your partner's complaints. It helps if you:

- Try to listen without interrupting.

- Make sure you understand your partner's feelings before formulating your response.

- Do not reflexively dismiss your partner's thoughts or feelings.

- Assume your partner's comments come from a place of love and caring. Accept the comments as an effort at strengthening your relationship.

- Trust that he or she wants to stay close and connected and that your behavior has been hurtful.

- Consider how difficult it is for your spouse to share these feelings with you.

- Recognize that it is often easier for a partner to choose resentment than honesty, so respect your partner's choice in talking with you. In the future, you will be grateful for the honesty.

ADDICTION

Addiction leads to another slippery slope. Abusing substances or engaging in harmful behaviors and dismissing your partner's concerns about it sends this message: my addiction is more important than my relationship. The most common substance addictions include alcohol, drugs, food, and tobacco. Addictive behaviors can include work, exercise, shopping, novelty-seeking, gambling, sex, pornography, video games, and the Internet or other technology. At best, addictive behaviors provide incomplete and short-term relief, but all addictive behavior leaves you worse off than you were before.

Many addictive behaviors are modes of self-soothing or self-medicating. The person may be anxious, depressed, scared, angry, grieving, or stressed. He or she may be trying to fill a void in his or her life. Engaging in addictive behaviors is frequently related to a desire to avoid feeling something painful, traumatic, or shameful. If the substance or damaging behavior is how you cope with painful emotions, being confronted by your partner about the issue may cause you to feel too exposed or vulnerable. From this perspective, it is understandable why a partner would be dismissive or avoidant with a spouse's concerns. But if the person who loves and cares for you most, who has made a lifetime commitment to be with you, believes that you might have a problem, it is important to listen. You may disagree with your partner's conclusion, and your partner may be incorrect in his or her assessment of the situation, but you still need to hear your partner's concerns.

Listening offers both of you an opportunity to find a way out of the woods.

Effective treatment of addictions often requires addressing the underlying thoughts, feelings, and emotions that trigger the behavior. No doubt, these are painful and sometimes shameful conversations to have with a partner. From my professional experience, many addictive behaviors affecting relationships go unaddressed for so long because they are difficult to introduce and discuss. Partners may be concerned that any discussion of a perceived addiction will be responded to with defensiveness or anger. However tempting it can be to ignore it, a real addiction that goes unaddressed will create chronic disengagement and unhappiness.

EXTRAMARITAL RELATIONSHIPS

It should not come as a surprise that long-term resentment leads to further problems, including infidelity. A partner who is not feeling loved, valued, appreciated, cared for, or heard may seek friendship, support, and affection from another. Ongoing resentment and emotional disconnection from one's partner can make both partners susceptible to seeking comfort from a work colleague, neighbor, another parent at school, or the high school friend you reconnected with on Facebook. From my clinical experience, infidelity in marriage most often starts with feeling disconnected, neglected, or dismissed by one's partner. If you are living with unaddressed resentment, anger, and unresolved conflict, your relationship is in danger.

While both partners may contribute to the context in which an affair occurs, emotional or sexual infidelity is a choice made by the unfaithful partner. It is a choice not to confront the distress in your marriage, and it is choosing to be distracted by the attraction to another. Confronting long-term unhappiness and disconnection in a marriage is not an easy undertaking. However, at best, infidelity only serves to complicate your life and your marriage. Never in my professional experience have I worked with partners who have regretted trying to reconnect or repair a relationship that has fractured from chronic resentment and emotional and physical disconnection. However, I have encountered numerous clients who deeply regretted participating in an affair that later precipitated a desperate attempt at reconnection or a painful divorce.

When a Facebook or other flirtation has gone so far as to threaten the foundation of your relationship and partner's trust, it is time to pause and seriously contemplate the risks inherent to this new relationship. If your spouse would be uncomfortable with your new friendship, take the necessary steps to protect yourself and your partner from future hurt and relational damage. By definition, infidelity is a slippery slope because extramarital relationships often escalate quickly. Remorse and regret surface just as quickly. Erase the other person's phone number. Do not meet him or her for coffee, drinks, or lunch. Do not respond to text messages. Diminish and, if possible, cut off all contact. This may be easier said than done. Accept all of these feelings as a sign that all is not right in your marriage. Your mutual commitment deserves a chance at rebuilding. Even if your attempts at marital repair fail, you will not regret trying.

IT MAY BE TIME TO SEEK HELP FROM A
MENTAL HEALTH PROFESSIONAL:

- If your partner regularly minimizes or dismisses your emotions or concerns, and you are feeling as though your partner does not listen to you.
- When anger and disrespect color your interactions.
- When you find yourself unable to move beyond resentment.
- If your partner is passive-aggressive—he or she says whatever it takes to avoid an argument but does nothing to fix the problem.
- When you cannot communicate respectfully or problem-solve effectively.
- When you realize there is an addiction to substances or behaviors that is interfering in your relationship and degrading the health of you or your partner.
- When your partner is overly negative and critical, and you stop listening to his or her complaints.
- When you do not feel appreciated or valued in your relationship.
- If you are feeling depressed or hopeless.
- If you think that your relationship cannot get better.
- When you or your partner seek support, friendship, or affection from someone outside of your marriage.

Slippery slopes can be sneaky, but they always involve a choice. You are in control of your marriage's future. The keys to avoid falling prey to a slippery slope within your relationship is to remain aware of common warning signs and keep the lines of communication open with your partner. Stay active in maintaining your relationship, and you are less likely to slide passively into resentment. It is often hardest to initiate a vulnerable conversation when you feel resentful or dismissed, but once you and your partner express mutual interest in rectifying your relationship, such conversation becomes habitual and more comfortable over time.

POINTS TO REMEMBER

- Commitment is a choice to maintain a healthy and honest connection with our partners.

- Before choosing resentment, choose communication.

- Strive to be attentive and caring, considerate and respectful, loving and kind, interested and interesting toward your partner.

- Recognize the importance of affection, connection, and gratitude as necessary aspects of keeping your relationship thriving.

- If your partner tells you that you are drinking, splurging, gambling, or online too much, listen to his or her concerns. Your partner knows you well and has noticed a change that he or she finds troubling. Even if you disagree with your partner's assessment, try to listen without getting defensive and angry.

- Recognize when you have become susceptible to an attractive distraction, and refocus on your partner.

- Before reconnecting with someone on social media or in person, discuss it with your partner.

For more resources, go to:

www.DrAnneMalec.com

CHAPTER TEN:

Forgiving and Repairing

Forgiveness is a requirement for a successful and happy marriage. We all screw up. We say the wrong thing, do the wrong thing, or are rude, inconsiderate, selfish, distracted, thoughtless, or maybe even mean-spirited. Many mistakes are unintentional, while others come from a place of wanting to hurt, make a point, be passive-aggressive, or because we are angry or resentful. No matter who said or did what, repairing relationship mistakes is fundamental to maintaining a strong connection to one's partner.

WHAT IS FORGIVENESS?

Forgiveness takes place in our minds and hearts. It is the deliberate decision to release oneself from feelings of resentment and a desire for vengeance against another. For many, it is not an easy emotional task to master because of the vulnerability it requires. Forgiveness does not mean the harmful behavior is excused or forgotten, nor does it require that another ask you for forgiveness. Forgiveness benefits the giver and the receiver, and it releases the hurt party from dedicating time and emotional resources to ruminating on the issue. Relationships lasting a lifetime continuously require intentional acts of forgiveness. Think of practicing forgiveness as building a muscle that keeps getting stronger with repetition.

Physical and Emotional Benefits of Forgiveness

Research informs us of the following benefits of forgiving:

- Healthier relationships
- Greater spiritual and psychological well-being
- Less anxiety, stress, and hostility
- Lower blood pressure
- Fewer symptoms of depression
- Stronger immune system
- Improved heart health
- Higher self-esteem[49]

Forgiveness is essential to the healing process after a hurt has occurred in the relationship. When you find yourself struggling to forgive yourself or your partner for a transgression, refer to these benefits and allow yourself to see the big picture. You and your partner are human, there will be mistakes, but successful marriages need to be flexible and adapt to these challenges.

Asking for Forgiveness

True expressions of apology and remorse require that the person at fault hold him or herself accountable for his or her words or actions. It will help your partner in the forgiveness process if you can honestly articulate the thoughts and emotions behind the hurtful action. Although it can be tempting to do so, it helps if you do not try to justify or rationalize your actions. Applying partial blame on your partner or giving qualified expressions of apology or remorse, such as "I am sorry if you took offense at my actions" also muddies the apology. Be clear and direct about what you are apologizing for, and express genuine remorse. Try to form an apology like this:

- I am sorry that I had too much to drink and embarrassed you in front of your parents. I will try to not do it again.

- I am sorry that my words were so painful to you. In hindsight, I realize I was distracted and failed to see how hurtful they could be.

- I am sorry for hanging up on you. I was frustrated by our conversation and just wanted it to end, but it was wrong of me to end it as I did.

If you apologize and your partner needs to talk more about it, do your best to avoid defensiveness or rejecting his or her request for further discussion. Frequently, the hurt partner will want to continue focusing on the harmful behavior because he or she is having trouble understanding what happened and why it happened. As the partner seeking forgiveness and feeling badly about what occurred, it is normal to want to limit or avoid feelings of shame and blame. However, resisting further discussion can create suspicion in the hurt partner or damage your attempts at repair. Be patient and try to empathize with your partner's difficulty in letting the issue go. Forgiveness is a gradual process.

Frustration can build if the apologizing partner feels as if the hurt partner is using the opportunity to pile on past failings or other wrongs. A suggestion for the hurt partner, do your best not to dump additional blame, as it discourages your partner's future repair attempts. To the partner seeking forgiveness, do your best to contain your frustration, as it will only serve to prolong the emotional repair process. Allow the hurt partner to process his or her feelings in a manner that allows space for understanding and closure.

What Does It Take to Forgive?

As previously stated, forgiveness is a gradual and non-linear process. Try to keep in mind that forgiveness requires action on the part of the forgiver to overcome feelings of hurt or anger toward the other partner. Additionally, forgiveness requires thoughtful consideration of the other's hurtful actions or words. Ask yourself, *Why did the words, actions, or inactions cause such hurt? Am I overly sensitive? How big of a deal was the infraction/hurt/slight? Was it an intentional act by my partner or just an oversight or mistake?* Remaining aware of your assumptions and sensitivities allows you to reach forgiveness with a clearer idea of your feelings for your partner and your hopes for your marriage's future.

You can aid forgiveness by attempting to put yourself in the other's shoes to understand what caused the harmful behavior. What does your partner have going on in his or her life? Could the hurtful behavior be related to being distracted with work or by a physical or emotional problem? Was the hurtful behavior a sign of an unaddressed or unresolved conflict? Was it passive-aggression? Were the words or actions related to feelings of resentment? If so, has your partner made previous unsuccessful attempts at bringing attention to the issues that have created the resentment? I do not mean to say that you are at fault for your partner causing you pain, but sometimes our self-protective instincts can prevent us from seeing the role we play in relationship problems. Regardless of the role you played in the transgression, empathy or putting yourself in the other's shoes is essential in accepting your partner's actions and moving forward.

Finally, you must act on your desire for forgiveness, which means you must resist the impulse to hold a grudge or retaliate, as doing this will only cause further pain in your relationship. If you genuinely desire forgiveness, you must play the part and create an environment for forgiveness to grow. To forgive means you have accepted that your partner engaged in a behavior that was hurtful to you, and you are choosing not to remain emotionally stuck in the negative space. Forgiveness benefits you, your partner, your marital bond, and your children. You forgive because you understand that you, too, have and will continue to require forgiveness.

Not every partner will ask for forgiveness, but he or she may still take actions to express his or her remorse or regret. You can choose to forgive without your partner asking for forgiveness. Try to not let the actions or inactions of your partner control your decision-making. The ability and willingness to forgive speaks to one's strength of character, relationship commitment, and emotional maturity.

Roadblocks to Forgiveness

For some partners, apologizing or expressing sorrow or remorse for hurtful actions creates anxiety and discomfort. Perhaps you know or *are* someone like this. Are you the type of person who finds it difficult to accept responsibility for hurting your partner? This reluctance for accountability can stem from wanting to avoid being in a one-down position; that is, by apologizing, you may feel that it creates an imbalance in the relationship by giving your partner more control. For some, admitting "you are right, and I am wrong" creates feelings of weakness or powerlessness. Admitting mistakes and taking responsibility for hurt feelings can cause a partner to feel uncomfortably vulnerable or emotionally at-risk. The thought process may look something like this: "If I admit to hurting my partner and apologize, he or she may determine that I am not worthy of forgiveness. He or she may see me as too flawed to continue to be in this relationship."

In the mind of this partner, apologizing implies that he or she encompasses flaws and imperfections and is potentially unlovable. If he or she is not lovable, his or her partner may leave. Thus, by denying or resisting the need for apology, the partner avoids the potential for all of this emotional unpleasantness. Even though the reluctance to apologize is understandable given the vulnerability it requires, it is still a poor relationship habit. Recognizing that we are worthy of love even with our flaws is one of the most rewarding aspects of a relationship. Give it a try. Ask for forgiveness, feel vulnerable, and trust that your partner will still love you, flaws and all.

On the other side of the coin, are you someone who resists forgiving others? Do you find yourself frequently ruminating over past hurts and keeping a running tally of your partner's wrongs? What keeps you stuck in this negative thought process? Do you withhold forgiveness from your partner because:

- You are concerned that forgiveness will only enable your partner to do it again?

- You lack an understanding of the event?

- It feels like you and your partner are in an ongoing hurt-and-forgiveness cycle?

- You are trying to make your partner feel shame?

- You are trying to maintain emotional distance in your relationship, that is, to protect yourself from closeness or vulnerability?

- The apology does not seem genuine?

- You want your partner to feel insecure in the relationship?

- You feel like you are always being wronged or hurt?

- Forgiveness means you deserved the poor treatment or that your spouse thinks poorly of you?

- The hurtful words or actions trigger a memory of abuse from childhood that pours salt on that early wound?

- You have a long-held, unaddressed resentment?

Many of the concerns mentioned above can create an unsafe emotional space in your relationship. If a partner feels that you cannot or will not let go of a hurt from the past no matter how much he or she apologizes, you are, in effect, pushing your partner away. If your partner feels that he or she never receives forgiveness for genuinely apologizing or if an apology only opens the door for piling on all his or her past mistakes or hurts, your partner may stop apologizing altogether. Just as in asking for forgiveness, offering forgiveness requires emotional courage and the trust that your partner will not manipulate or take advantage of your vulnerability.

If you find yourself struggling to forgive your partner, you are no doubt aware that it is damaging to your marriage. A therapist can help. Sometimes an inability to forgive a partner stems from a lack of trust in others, your partner included. You may feel as though those who profess to love you frequently wrong you. It is not unusual for a lack of trust in others to develop from an insecure and unstable relationship with a primary caregiver, such as a parent. If this is you, talking to a mental health professional will help you gain clarity about these feelings and experiences.

Dedicating emotional and mental space to anger or the nursing of a grudge is hurtful to you and pushes away your partner.

Forgiving our partners for their mistakes sends the message that we can empathize and accept their flaws, and it helps set the stage for when we, too, will need forgiveness. It is critically important to the health of a relationship that genuine apologies are given and accepted.

FOR THE PARTNER SEEKING FORGIVENESS THAT NEVER SEEMS TO COME.

It is okay to respectfully express your frustration when your attempts at repair get continuously rebuffed. Communicate your frustration to your partner about his or her seeming unwillingness to forgive after you have expressed genuine remorse for your words or actions. If your partner denies your apologies or does not recall you offering one, apologize again and ask for forgiveness. Ask the hurt partner what he or she needs to hear from you in order to move on. If the answer is "I don't know," no doubt you will continue to feel frustration and perhaps anger. However, frustration expressed as anger will backfire on you. Much of the time, your partner genuinely does not know what he or she needs to hear or feel to be willing to offer forgiveness and may need more time to understand and process the event.

Let your partner know that you genuinely want to know what steps to take to earn forgiveness. Without knowing what your partner needs to accept your apology and offer forgiveness, there will continue to be frustration and hurt in the relationship. It is important to let your partner know when you feel discouraged or frustrated, but it is essential to show your partner that you are committed to repairing the relationship. For the reluctant forgiver: Be mindful that after multiple attempts at earning forgiveness, some partners give up trying altogether.

SEEMINGLY UNFORGIVEABLE ACTS

I do not address in this book acts of domestic violence or physical abuse that occur within a relationship. For many, these actions are unforgivable and often require outside assistance to achieve safety to have any hope of repairing the relationship. The sense of betrayal and shattered trust stemming from abuse is often insurmountable and destroys the relationship. Another form of relationship betrayal that is often difficult to forgive is infidelity. The next section addresses this topic.

REPAIRING INFIDELITY

Repairing a relationship after infidelity is one of the most difficult processes any couple can face. The pain, hurt, devastation, sadness, anger, sense of betrayal, and shame can feel overwhelming. You may have found yourself completely shocked by the revelation—or perhaps, not shocked at all, because your intuition was telling you something was not quite right in your relationship. In the time immediately following the affair exposure, both partners are usually in a panic but for different reasons. The hurt partner can feel as though his or her life has been completely turned upside down because the person he or she trusted more than anyone else committed a betrayal. The unfaithful partner is often trying to calm the angry and hurt partner while also managing guilt and grief over the loss of the extramarital relationship.

What Causes Infidelity?

Many factors can contribute to infidelity, but common ones are long-term emotional and physical disconnection, depression, feeling neglected or unheard, and anger or resentment. However, not everyone who cheats is unhappy in the marriage: sometimes it occurs because a partner becomes susceptible to feeling "special" again. He or she liked knowing that another found him or her attractive, flirting felt good, or maybe the partner was bored or disenchanted with life. Perhaps he or she could not deny the attraction, rationalized that it would only be once and not hurt anyone, or maybe the partner acted while intoxicated. While it it usually true that both partners are responsible for relational disrepair, the blame for infidelity falls squarely on the shoulders of the unfaithful.

For the Hurt Partner:

The emotional swings a hurt partner experiences after the affair is revealed can feel dizzying and earth-shattering. Because being faced with the betrayal of infidelity can make you feel powerless, you may feel an overwhelming desire to do *something*. You might feel that the unfaithful partner should leave the home temporarily or move out permanently. You may want to immediately contact an attorney and declare your desire for a divorce, transfer funds from a joint account, and tell family, friends, neighbors, or even employers about the affair.

While these emotional reactions are completely understandable in the immediate aftermath of the affair exposure, you will probably feel differently in a week and will definitely feel differently in a month. As tempting as it is, you should avoid making impulsive decisions that feel right in the moment but only serve to damage your relationship and personal well-being further. As difficult as it can feel to *not do something* that shows the depth of your hurt and anger, it may be wise to wait a few weeks or a few months before making significant decisions about your future. Giving yourself this time allows you to think and feel your way to more clear-headed choices. However, you should seek distance and safety if you believe that either you or your partner is at risk for physical harm or violence.

Determining what you want and how best to proceed can be achieved only through creating time and space for understanding and emotional processing. To remain resilient and stable during the days and weeks after the exposure, consider doing some of the following:

- Contact and make an appointment with a qualified and licensed therapist.

- Confide in a friend or family member who you know is loyal and loving to both you and your partner and will continue to support you no matter what you decide.

- Engage in self-care aimed at reducing stress: yoga, massage, leisurely walks in the sunshine, meditation, and spending time with some of your favorite people.

- Get outside and walk, run, cycle...move and get some exercise.

- Try to maintain a normal routine for your children. They do not need to know and should not know about infidelity in their parents' relationship.

- Try to accept and tolerate your mood swings. These are normal to the circumstances and will gradually subside.

- You may not feel hungry, but it is important to eat and receive nutrition.

- Try to stay socially engaged with friends, work, and social activities.

- Be aware of how much alcohol you are consuming, and do not allow it to become your means of self-soothing.

- If you have a strong faith, pray for wisdom and patience.

For the Unfaithful Partner:

When a partner learns of infidelity, it can feel like the person that he or she loves and trusts the most has literally and figuratively knocked the wind out of him or her. The hurt partner will be angry, scared, and sad. The anger you feel from your partner may come in waves; emotions can and do turn very quickly. Your partner's life has been turned upside down. Your partner is in pain, and, unfortunately, you caused that pain. Your instinct may be to hide or dispose of incriminating evidence that will further hurt your partner. You want to avoid making it worse than it already is, but any hope of relationship repair requires that you remain open and honest with your partner from here on out.

Once an affair is in the open, your partner will start to second-guess and question your past conversations, trips, absences, late nights, strange explanations, and so on. You may have gotten into the habit of lying or being elusive or noncommittal with your partner, but for your relationship to have a chance at recovering, the lying must stop. All of us have a self-protective instinct that evolved to keep us safe. After the affair comes to light, this instinct may shift into overdrive for both of you. For the hurt partner, it means doing everything in his or her power to determine if you are telling the truth, often leading to the same questions about aspects of the affair over and over. For you, it may seem tempting to fudge or omit details in order to lessen the damage and hurt manifested by the truth. However, recognize that continuing to lie will only serve to delay the repair and rebuilding process.

For there to be a chance at healing the relationship, the hurt partner needs to understand exactly what happened and why it happened. This knowledge is used to build a narrative of under-standing and to absorb and process what happened. Without a coherent narrative, there will continue to be nagging doubts and questions about the events. If your partner's instinct leads him or her to question your explanations or inconsistencies, he or she may look further by searching for a paper, phone, website, or text message trail. The questions asked of the unfaithful partner might seem repetitive and constant, but they are necessary for understanding. Come clean. I have seen couples struggle for years in trying to piece together the full story because the unfaithful partner resists answering questions and providing details. Often, the unfaithful partner will try to cover up or lie after the affair is exposed, only for the truth to come out later, often from the sleuthing of the hurt partner. Trust is much more difficult to rebuild after a relationship breach than it was initially, so be patient with your partner's recovery process.

Another common mistake made by an unfaithful spouse is to blame a partner for the affair. In a desperate attempt to explain or rationalize infidelity, the unfaithful partner will claim it is a result of feeling neglected by his or her partner. The hurt partner may be blamed for not being interested in having sex, working too much, always being angry, drinking too much, or failing to meet a partner's emotional needs. While any and all of these reasons may be true in creating the context in which the affair occurred, it does not excuse a partner's infidelity. An unfaithful partner should never take the approach of blaming his or her partner for com-mitting an affair, because that was still a choice solely made by the unfaithful partner. I understand how the unfaithful partner can be tempted to project blame onto the spouse: his or her feelings of shame and guilt need an outlet. Unfaithful partners attempt to justify the unjustifiable, and it can feel emotionally overwhelming to admit the size of this error in judgment to themselves and their partners.

To repair the relationship, you must be honest, patient, and genuinely remorseful of the pain you have caused. Genuine remorse does not include self-pity or trying to manipulate your partner into feeling badly for you because of the shame you feel about your actions. This is the time to focus on your partner, be truthful, take responsibility, and begin the trust rebuilding process, which will take longer than you hope.

Communicating with your partner about the infidelity is where the hard emotional repair work starts. While you may not be able to clearly articulate the reasons for the affair or what was missing from your marriage or your life, you can be sure that there are reasons that led you astray. The reasons might be tough to talk about, but no doubt about it, there are reasons. The work of emotional repair starts with self-reflection, honest conversations with your partner, couple therapy, and individual therapy. Your partner wants to trust you, so give him or her a reason to do so.

As long as there are people in a relationship, there will be mistakes. It is impossible to avoid hurting your partner throughout the entirety of a marriage. Whether it is smaller transgressions like forgetting to call home when you will be late from work or larger betrayals like infidelity, your relationship will encounter obstacles that necessitate forgiveness and repair for the relationship to move forward. It can be an arduous process, but it is one both partners must commit to when they take their vows.

POINTS TO REMEMBER

- Apologies and expressions of remorse require honesty, genuineness, and accountability.

- Forgiveness is a requirement in a loving relationship.

- Asking for and offering forgiveness requires trust in your partner and a willingness to be vulnerable.

- Stubbornly refusing to apologize or forgive will have damaging consequences to the health of your relationship.

- Forgiveness is a gift you give to yourself, your partner, your relationship, and your children.

- Infidelity is a profound breach of trust in a marriage and has consequences.

- If your partner cheats on you and you discover it, do not act in haste to make sweeping changes in your life. Your perspective will change over the days, weeks, and months ahead.

- Seek help from a qualified therapist to work through the issues infidelity creates.

- If you are the partner who cheated, be prepared to deal with your hurt partner's justifiable anger, pain, and outrage. Do not deflect it by blaming your infidelity on your partner.

- After an affair, trust is rebuilt through a slow and consistent process of engaging in trustworthy behaviors. Think of it as making daily deposits in the trust bank.

For more resources, go to:
www.DrAnneMalec.com

CONCLUSION

Marriage is an ancient institution, but modern marriages face complex obstacles that did not historically exist. Partners today must communicate openly, nourish their emotional connection, and tackle the stress of modern life as a team. You and your partner will make mistakes and experience conflict, but through using the tools in this book, you will be better prepared to remedy your mistakes and find compromise.

A few final thoughts to keep in mind for preserving all that drew you together in the first place:

- Humans evolved to habituate to our circumstances, but daily sameness in marriage can feel boring. Partners must commit to remaining interesting to their spouses. Ask yourself: How do I keep my relationship fresh? How do I maintain some level of mystery? How do we maintain interest in each other? It may help to recall specifically what initially drew you to your partner and what drew him or her to you. How did you try to impress your partner? Do not stop doing the things that made you attractive to him or her. And make sure your partner is aware of how much he or she means to you every day.

- Find shared activities that you both enjoy. Be ready to compromise—to engage in something your spouse loves even if you do not—because such efforts nurture your love. Maintaining a solid emotional connection and friendship requires active dedication.

- Have healthy and frequent communications, including a weekly check-in and date night. Tell your mate that you love him or her daily. Kiss and hug your partner every day, multiple times. Express gratitude, appreciation, and validation as often as you want to hear it yourself!

- It is important that the couple relationship remains a priority, especially as it conflicts with other responsibilities, such as work and parenting. Adults today can easily become wrapped up in their children at the cost of their marriages. Discuss your expectations, concerns, and hopes regarding parenting. Even in this day and age, the father can wind up feeling like second best, so make sure you share parent work and joy together. But since your marriage is important to your children as well as you, remember to keep your relationship a priority. If parents can take care of their intimate relationship, the children will flourish.

- Few modern couples are properly prepared for sharing household economic decisions. Talk about your financial goals and expectations openly with your partner, and set an agreed-upon financial arrangement for your family. Remember to check in regularly to ensure the arrangement is still working for both of you. Ensure your budget includes a reasonable personal monthly budget for each of you that is not subject to the partner's input.

- Sex is a vital aspect of satisfying relationships. It is normal for sexual desire to fluctuate over time, so be sure you create a conversational safety zone to enable talk about this sensitive and important issue.

- Resentment is a slippery slope. If either of you have a problem in your relationship, choose to face it rather than allow resentment to come between you, as it surely will. Work with your partner to create a safe space to talk about relationship hurts and concerns. Do not be afraid to seek professional assistance if you find you or your partner struggling to close the distance between you.

- Forgiveness is essential to long-term relationships. Remain aware of your sensitivities and obstacles to forgiveness. Apologize and own your mistakes. Listen to what your partner needs from you to achieve forgiveness.

In summary, a spouse must be someone you can count on, both a partner and a romantic attraction. With all our modern duties and distractions, it can be easy to take this person, and all they mean to us, for granted. But, as your most important asset, you must care for and nurture your love.

For those struggling to master the challenges of a long-term relationship, I hope this book provides the assistance you need to help your marriage thrive. Marriage is a choice and a commitment to uphold vows based on your beliefs, goals, and priorities. Do not lose sight of the importance of this relationship. Vow to each other to be successful spouses in this modern life.

NOTE TO READERS:

If you would like to receive updates about this book or any future books, would like to provide feedback, or would like to participate in relationship surveys, please visit

www.DrAnneMalec.com.

ENDNOTES

1   Centers for Disease Control and Prevention. "National survey of family growth." *CDC,* September 3, 2013. http://www.cdc.gov/nchs/nsfg/key_statistics/d.htm#divorce (accessed February 20, 2015).

2   Lynn Gigy and Joan B. Kelly. "Perspectives on divorcing men and women." *Journal of Divorce and Remarriage,* 1993: 169-188.

3   A.J. Hawkins, B.J Willoughby, and W.J. Doherty, "Reasons for divorce and openness to marital reconciliation," *Journal of Divorce and Remarriage* (2012): 453-463.

4   Scott Coltrane and Randall Collins. *Sociology of Marriage and the Family.* Belmont: Wadsworth, 2001.

5   *About Schmidt.* Directed by Alexander Payne, 2002.

6   Clint Black, "Something That We Do." Comps. C. Black and S. Ewing, 1997.

7   Andrew K. Przybylski and Netta Weinstein. "Can you connect with me now? How the presence of mobile communication technology influences face-to-face conversation quality." *Journal of Social and Personal Relationships,* 2012: 237-246.

8   Brandon T. McDaniel and Sarah M. Coyne. "Technoference: the interference of technology in couple relationships and implications for women's personal and relational well-being." *Psychology of Popular Media Culture,* 2014.

9   *The Economist.* "Planet of the phones." February 28, 2015: 9.

10 "The 5 Love Languages" website. http://www.5lovelanguages.com/ (accessed February 09, 2015).

11 E. Hatfield and R.L. Rapson, "Equity theory in close relationships." In *Handbook of Theories of Social Psychology*, by A.W. Kruglanski, E.T. Higgins, and P.A.M. Van Lange, eds. (pp. 200-217). London: Glyph International, 2011.

12 John Gottman. *Why Marriages Succeed or Fail.* Simon and Schuster, 1995.

13 "Families with own children: Employment status of parents by age of youngest child and family type, 2012-2013 annual averages." Bureau of Labor Statistics, last modified April 23, 2015, www.bls.gov: http://www.bls.gov/news.release/famee.t04.htm.

14 Sylvia Ann Hewlett and Carolyn Buck Lace, "Off-Ramps and On-Ramps: Keeping Talented Women on the Road to Success," *Harvard Business Review*, March 2005, https://hbr.org/2005/03/off-ramps-and-on-ramps-keeping-talented-women-on-the-road-to-success/ar/1.

15 Ibid.

16 Ann Critenden, *The Price of Motherhood.* (New York: Picador, 2010).

17 Suzanne M. Bianchi, Lekha Subaiya, and Joan R. Kah, "The Gender Gap and Economic Well-Being of Non-Resident Fathers and Custodial Mothers," *Demography* 36 (1999): 196-203.

18 Melanie Hicken, "Why many retired women live in poverty," CNN Money, last modified May 13, 2014, http://money.cnn.com/2014/05/13/retirement/retirement-women.

19 Karen Z. Kramer and Jan B. McColloch. "Stay at home fathers: definitions and characteristics based on 42 years of CPS data."

Population Association of America: Annual meeting in Dallas, Texas. 2010.

20 Gretchen Livingston. "Growing number of dads home with the kids." *Pew Research Center.* June 5, 2014. http://www.pewsocial-trends.org/2014/06/05/growing-number-of-dads-home-with-the-kids/ (accessed March 7, 2015).

21 Wendy Wang, Kim Parker, and Paul Taylor. "Breadwinner moms." *Pew Research Center: Social and Demographic Trends.* May 29, 2013. http://www.pewsocialtrends.org/2013/05/29/breadwinner-moms/ (accessed February 19, 2015).

22 N. Chesley, "Stay-at-home fathers and breadwinning mothers," *Gender and Society* (2011): 642-664.

23 "Labor force statistics from the current population survey." *Bureau of Labor Statistics.* March 24, 2012. http://www.bls.gov/cps/wives_earn_more.htm (accessed February 24, 2015).

24 Veronica Tichener, "Maintaining men's dominance: negotiating identity and power when she earns more." *Sex Roles*, 2005: 191-205.

25 Marianne Bertrand, Emir Kamenica, and Jessica Pan. "Gender identity and relative income within households." http://faculty.chicagobooth.edu/emir.kamenica/documents/identity.pdf, 2012.

26 Torabi, Farnoosh. *When She Makes More: 10 Rules for Breadwinning Women.* Penguin Publishing Group, 2014.

27 National Endowment for Financial Education. "The extramarital bank account: tales of financial infidelity." *Chicago Tribune*, February 15, 2015.

28 American Academy of Matrimonial Lawyers. "Increase of prenuptial agreements reflects improving economy and real estate market: survey of nation's top matrimonial attorneys also cites rise in women

requesting prenups." October 15, 2013. http://www.aaml.org/
about-the-academy/press/press-releases/pre-post-nuptial-agreements/
increase-prenuptial-agreements-re (accessed February 16, 2015).

29 "Stepfamily fact sheet." *National Stepfamily Resource Center.*
February 27, 2015. http://www.stepfamilies.info/stepfamily-fact-
sheet.php (accessed February 27, 2015).

30 Chrisanna Northrup, Pepper Schwartz, and James Witte. *The
Normal Bar: The Surprising Secrets of Happy Couples and What
They Reveal About Creating a New Normal in Your Relation-
ship.* New York: Harmony Books, 2012.

31 Stuart Brody. "The relative health benefits of different sexual
activities." *Journal of Sexual Medicine*, 2010: 1336-1361.

32 *Health and Sex.* n.d. http://www.webmd.com/sex-relationships/
guide/sex-and-health?page=2 (accessed February 21, 2015).

33 Ibid.

34 Ibid.

35 Ibid.

36 Ibid.

37 Sarah Murray and Robin Milhausen. "Factors impacting women's
sexual desire: examining long-term relationships in emerging
adulthood." *The Canadian Journal of Human Sexuality*, 2012.

38 Esther Perel. *The secret to desire in a long term relationship*
(February 2013).

39 Mayo Clinic Staff. "Female sexual dysfunction." September 25,
2012. http://www.mayoclinic.org/diseases-conditions/female-sex-
ual-dysfunction/basics/definition/con-20027721 (accessed March
11, 2015).